THE HORMONE SHIFT

THE HORMONE SHIFT

USING NATURAL HORMONE BALANCING FOR YOUR
Mood, Weight, Sleep & Female Health

DAWN M. CUTILLO

Ordering Information:

For orders and inquiries, please contact:
1-888-375-9818
www.toplinkpublishing.com
bookorder@toplinkpublishing.com

Printed in the United States of America

My heartfelt thanks to all my clients over the years who supported me and believed in my efforts to change the way we look at weight loss and hormone balancing.

I also would like to thank our growing network of franchisees. These people have dedicated their time and efforts to start BeBalanced Hormone Weight Loss Centers to aid me in promoting the benefits of Natural Hormone Balancing!

Ten sure-fire Signs that your Hormones have *Shifted*. . .

1. Everyone around you needs an attitude adjustment.

2. You can't understand why chocolate isn't on the food guide pyramid.

3. You find yourself counting flocks of sheep and you still can't sleep!

4. You find yourself using your cell phone to dial up every bumper sticker that says, *"How's my driving? Call* 1-800 . . ." to give your opinion!

5. You are eating less than your 11 year old child and still can't seem to lose a pound!

6. Your husband has decided it's better to agree with everything that you say.

7. The dry cleaner has definitely shrunk every last pair of your pants.

8. Wine is no longer a weekend treat but a daily staple . . . *at lunch!*

9. Your pesky PMS symptoms are now part of your everyday life.

10. Your nights are now filled with "hot flashes" instead of "hot sex."

CONTENTS

FOREWORD

I am so pleased to be able to write a foreword for Dawn Cutillo's book, The Hormone Shift , because some of my very own clients have made huge improvements in their lives as a result of using her services. Furthermore, I have had the opportunity to watch Dawn herself benefit in every way by using and living by the healthy, natural choices that she promotes. Dawn's work at her local center and her research for this book are unique in that her emphasis is on the importance of hormones and their effect on every part of the body, which in turn affects the mind and the spirit.

Our work connects on a deep level because I have spent the majority of my fifty-five year career being concerned with the way that the mind affects the body and spirit. Similarly, Dawn's training and interest have been primarily in the area of physical health and the way in which the health of the body affects the mind and general well-being. Our paths cross over sharing common interest in the intersection of psychology, religion and healing. We find common ground in that we share the belief that the body, mind and spirit are intertwined, and that what affects one, affects the whole. We both believe that "dis-ease" can lead to disease. Our work seems to complement each other. Dawn begins with the body and its effect on the mind and spirit—my work begins with psychological concerns, which in turn affect a person's general health and well being. My work as a stress management consultant and psychology teacher, coupled with my fifty-five years in private practice (specializing in psychotherapy, dream work, and couples counseling) gives me unique insight into matters of the psyche and their direct affect on physiology. After meeting Dawn and learning of her work, I found a bridge between the mind-body connection. I visited her health center many years ago and availed myself of some of her services.

A little about my background . . .

My education began with a BA degree in Religion with a minor in Psychology, which was later followed by a Master's Degree in Counseling Psychology and a Doctorate in Psychology—the latter two from Temple University. My postdoctoral degree in Cognitive Psychology was acquired through the University of Pennsylvania. I finished my professional career at Elizabeth town College, in Elizabeth town, PA where I served as the college chaplain and the Psychological Consultant to the Counseling Center. Over the years I have worked in the court system in both Harrisburg, PA and London, England. My husband and I operated a large Children's Home through the London County Council, followed by work with delinquent boys at the Casa Della Scugnizzi in Naples, and then back to Trenton State College (now College of New Jersey) where we both served on the faculty. Over the years I have taught undergraduate Psychology at the State University of New York, Franklin and Marshall College and Elizabeth town College. I have also taught graduate coursework in Adult Developmental Psychology at Temple University and Penn State University.

My interest in stress and stress management began thirty-five years ago when I read the research of Hans Selye, M.D., a Canadian researcher, who first studied the effect of stress on every organ in the body, which at that time was a revolutionary concept. This coincided with my discovery of the whole new field of relaxation techniques and of meditation, which could reduce stress and influence healing. I was the Stress Management Consultant for the Office of Personnel Management, both Philadelphia and New York Regions. I developed a tape of relaxation techniques and an introduction to meditation, which I included in my handouts. Over the years at various colleges and universities I also gave out relaxation tapes to students, especially at exam time. I continued to run workshops when I moved to Lancaster County.

Throughout the years, my job took me to many locations and through many approaches to human services, which only reinforced my understanding that all persons, male and female, adult and child and from various cultures share the same physical, psychological, personal and spiritual needs and concerns. We share, not only the same blood, but also as Carl Jung discovered, the same psychological architecture of the brain/mind. My doctoral dissertation was on the work of Dr. Carl Jung who was the first psychologist to talk about the importance of man's spiritual nature. I studied at the Jung Institute then located in Zurich, Switzerland. Jung brought together for me the fields of psychology, religion and healing.

It is interesting to note that the questions about human purpose and health were first the province of Religion; it later evolved into Philosophy and out of Philosophy came Psychology. Modern psychology claims both mind and spirit, recognizing that we are psychophysical beings with a need for purpose and meaning, the province of the spirit. The medical community now acknowledges this interconnectedness through the latest science: Psychoneuroimmunology; Psyche, the Greek word for Soul/ Mind, Neuro—the Neurological system, Immunology, the effect of personality on both the neurological system and the immune system. This is the fastest growing field of study in many of the major universities. I feel that work with balancing hormones is important as it will affect not only the physical body and aid those symptoms but will also positively affect the mind and spirit, and in turn affect all aspects of the total person.

At Dawn's center she recognizes all of the elements that create a total person. She is an expert on hormones, but in addition to the natural hormone therapies that she promotes, her center also provides an excellent weight loss program, relaxation therapy, natural supplements, nutritional counseling, massage, lymph drainage, Reiki and other services to promote overall education, relaxation and healing. This is a truly holistic approach. Another thing that impressed me about Dawn is that she highly believes in the role of stress management in overall health and hormonal balance. She produced an effective relaxation program for her clients, which included the latest "sound-wave" therapy now available due to the latest technology.

To me, the best advertisement for her center and her research is Dawn herself. Lovely to begin with, I have seen her lose weight arriving at an ideal size and maintaining it. Additionally, her skin condition, which erupted on occasion, has completely cleared, her spiritual work has made her more centered and she glows with enthusiasm and love for her work, which is truly her mission in life.

Patricia Joan Austin, Ph.D.

INTRODUCTION

W hy is it that women's fluctuating hormones are a frequent topic of discussion? Maybe it is because our hormone levels seem to define us through the various stages of life, as we each fight our own private battle with their effects. Each stage brings along with it its own shift until we finally reach the *big* shift that we term "menopause," or which seems to those approaching it, another word for *death!*

From puberty onward, we face the struggles and challenges of rapid physical and mental changes, followed by the monthly annoyance of premenstrual syndrome (PMS), then perhaps pregnancy and the possibility of experiencing postpartum depression. As we move into later adulthood, we begin the seemingly endless stages of pre-menopause and peri-menopause, and finally the potentially "catastrophic" experience of menopause itself. Each of these life stages brings a host of physical, mental, and emotional challenges that we must face—*all thanks to our hormones.*

Simply stated, hormones are chemicals that tell our cells what to do. In reality, hormones often seem like an enemy's army in our bodies that cause us to feel imbalanced, and at times, completely out of control! Even though these hormonal changes and their effects are often considered "female" problems, the symptoms associated with hormonal fluctuations certainly also provide daily difficulties for everyone around us; including our spouses, families, coworkers, and friends. In short, *no one* is immune to the incredible power of hormones!

There can even be controversy over how (or if) to bring our hormones into balance due to the varying measures that are taken to "fix" the issues. When considering what to do, many questions arise, such as: Which symptoms are "normal" and simply need to be managed? What symptoms might indicate a serious problem? Should we mask symptoms with the birth control pill? Is it okay to skip monthly periods? Should we supplement our hormones? Are synthetic hormones helpful or are they harmful? Are certain hormones safe for long-term use? What about bio -identical hormones? Are natural therapies really effective? Should we have our hormone levels tested? If so, which tests are best and produce the most accurate results?

I am writing this book with the intention to provide you with information on the cause of the hormonal shift and the problem that this shift can create at any age or stage of life, and then to discuss the current market solutions as well as the newly available solution of "natural hormone balancing." This should better enable you to make an educated decision as to what will be the safest and most effective path for you to take that works with your lifestyle. I do this while shining light on the controversy surrounding the topic of hormones in order to arm you with all of the available information. Having information puts you in control of your life and allows you to move through each phase of your life with ease and positive expectations.

Education is the key to understanding the basics of the female sex hormones (estrogen and progesterone) and the stress hormone (cortisol). What we do, how we think, and what we eat all have an effect on the production and levels of these hormones, as well as their conversion from one to another. In other words, you cannot totally avoid "Shift s" in hormones that come with some of the major stages of life but you do play a role in your own hormonal balance and can minimize any subsequent symptoms. This responsibility also gives you some control but certainly is not meant to place blame on you for your fluctuating hormones.

Bringing hormones into their natural balance and alleviating the symptoms of imbalances is not a task that general practitioners have perfected. Moreover, there is a plethora of conflicting information surrounding this field of study. One source will tell you that as we age we need estrogen for bone health, but then you may read elsewhere that estrogen is linked to certain cancers. So, what are we to think? It seems like the word "hormone" can conjure up scary images because hormones are often linked to certain cancers or hormone-sensitive tumors. This fear is also increased because of the lack of understanding and the poor education that is provided to women through the varying stages of life. There seems to be a mystery about how hormones work and how they interact with each other, so most people understandably think that it may be something that you do not want to tamper with. Many women, and even some doctors, are unsure of the risks of hormone replacement therapy, so they opt to just leave things alone. Others decide to push for some real answers. They want to know how their bodies work, desire to live symptom free, and look their best as they age.

I was one of the latter and my personal quest to understand what was going on with my body began when I was twelve. I suffered from crippling menstrual cramps that were so painful they kept me out of school. Getting out of class was no "Ferris Bueller's Day Off!" Instead, I was stuck at home rolling around in bed in intense pain. I later learned that this monthly affliction had a direct relationship with hormone balance, or more accurately; *imbalance.* Throughout the remainder of my teens and early twenties, I continued to suffer from hormone-related issues such as acne, fluid retention, and weight gain. Intuitively, I knew that something about my body was off (this was one of the factors that led me into the health field 30 years ago). I pursued my bachelor's degree in health and physical education and later became further educated in the fields of fitness, nutrition, detoxification, energy work, and finally hormonal balancing. Each of these was a stepping-stone to the next course of study, and my passion now lies in helping my clients balance their hormones so that they may control their symptoms, as well as reach and maintain a healthy weight.

About sixteen years ago, I met a certified clinical nutritionist from California, who is now a naturopathic doctor. He and his colleagues performed more than 20,000 saliva tests in the process of product development while starting a hormone testing lab, which is now one of the largest saliva testing facilities in the United States. The purpose was to offer natural hormone solutions and hormone testing to the public, as well as educate healthcare professionals. He possessed an in-depth understanding of the interactions between sex hormones and stress hormones, which is essential information for correctly balancing hormones. We worked together for several years doing saliva testing and consultations in order to aid women in balancing their hormones naturally. We even did national consulting and lecturing on the topic of "weight loss and hormones." A few years ago, in collaboration with another doctor, we performed a small breast cancer research study that was tabulated by the director of research at West Chester University (see Appendix B). This small study helped me to have further hands-on experience in learning about hormone interactions and to understand the foundation of hormone balance.

While I do not offer the final word on hormones, I hope I can serve as a voice of reason in the chaos of the conflicting information about hormones and their effects on our bodies. You will come to see by further reading that my approach on hormone balancing is the most conservative and safe approach while yielding fast, measurable results. My education is not from a book, as I feel experience is a much better teacher. My knowledge comes from first-hand experience observing before and after hormone saliva test results, performing my own hormone saliva tests on my own clients, and from my current experience working with thousands of women who achieve quick, safe, and natural results for their hormone-related problems.

In writing this book, I have included some documented sources and pertinent studies to verify certain facts, but I do not list pages upon pages of references. Interested parties who choose to do their own research will find that the type of natural hormone therapy specifically addressed in this book is virtually without side effects. In my practice, I mainly follow and employ some basics of the late John R. Lee, M.D.'s groundbreaking work in the field of natural progesterone therapy. However, I also take this a step further by addressing adrenal therapy while adding in information on nutrition, stress management and other lifestyle factors.

This book has nine chapters that fit into three basic sections. Although some chapters may not apply to a certain demographic (for example, a young woman may not wish to read about menopause), it would be wise to read the book in its entirety to get the full picture—even if you feel certain chapters or sections may not pertain to your stage of life. In the first section (Chapter 1), I cover the basics of hormones so that you can begin reading with a general understanding of what's going on with your body and generally how your hormones can "Shift." Following this basic discussion, we will go on to the second section and learn about how our hormonal shift s can cause imbalances in six different areas. With this I will discuss various therapies for your symptoms, as well as shed light on some controversial information. In Chapter 2, I will discuss the hormone shift and menopause, and the risks of traditional hormone replacement therapy; including synthetic and bio-identical hormones. In Chapter 3, which was totally revised in this revised edition, I will discuss the hormone shift and weight, and how using a protocol consisting of a low calorie ketogenic diet coupled with glandulars can aid in rapid and effective weight loss for women struggling with stubborn weight. In Chapter 4, I will look at the hormone shift and the thyroid gland; the tradition of using medications to treat thyroid symptoms. In Chapter 5, I will examine the hormone Shift and PMS; the newly popular "solution" of using the birth control pill to relieve PMS symptoms. In Chapter 6, I will touch on the hormone shift and mood; the traditional use of strong psychotropic medication to aid mood issues (depression/anxiety). In Chapter 7, I will discuss the hormone shift and aging; the use of HGH to slow the rapid aging process brought on by our modern world. In the last section of this book, Chapter 8, I will go over natural, safe and effective solutions that positively impact all of these areas. This will provide you with the necessary tools and information that will help to solve any issues relating to your weight, mood and overall health. Chapter 9 is a new addition to this revised book and shows how hair loss/thinning is effected directly by hormones and other lifestyle factors which can be adjusted for hair rejuvenation even as we age. Hair loss/ thinning has become an increasing large epidemic amount women, even though it is talked about more in reference to men. I felt deeper research was needed and I uncovered hormonal components and other factors that I have not read anywhere else as of yet.

Finding hormonal balance improved my life, and with the information in this book, I want to help you improve your life. I want to free you from the excess physical and emotional weight that you have been burdened with, so that you can become all you are meant to be. It is hard to find inner peace, true joy, self-actualization, and deep spiritual growth when you are living with the symptoms associated with out-of-balance hormones.

By the release of this revised edition, I will have helped not only thousands of women in my local area in Pennsylvania but hundreds all over the country who have read the first edition of this book after seeing me on some national daytime television shows I was privileged to appear on. This made me realize that women are the same everywhere, with the same hormone issues and life struggles and they all can be helped with natural hormone balancing. Natural hormone balancing is really just the process of having things go back to the way they were intended, no real magic is needed, we can just learn to work with the body and not against it.

My deepest desire is for you to not be weighed down by hormonal symptoms any longer, but rather, enjoy the fact that you are a woman! I believe the information in this book will resonate with you when you contemplate and internalize it. The reason, just like with thousands of other women, is because you already knew it...deep inside. Your intuition told you something was "off" and you knew things should not have to be this way. This information may be what you have been waiting for—or praying for—all along. Whenever I receive advice or new information that makes sense, I use my intuition and meditate or pray on it to see if it is truth. Truth will surface, as it always does . . . and when it does, *you will surely agree* with the biblical passage, "The truth will set you free."

CHAPTER 1

The Hormone Shift &
How it Affects Your Body

L et us start with Hormones 101, or the basics, to set the foundation for the rest of the book. Once you understand the basics of the sex and stress hormones, you will then be able to understand why balance is so important in order to avoid the symptoms of PMS, perimenopause, and menopause.

This book discusses in detail three of the major hormones: estrogen, progesterone, and cortisol. However, because all hormones have an important role in the body, I also touch upon some of the other hormones: follicle-stimulating hormone (FSH), luteinizing hormone (LH), testosterone, thyroid hormones (T3, T4 and TSH), DHEA, pregnenolone, melatonin, insulin, and Human Growth Hormones (HGH).

The process of how hormones are orchestrated in the body is delicate and complex, relying on a system of checks and balances in the form of feedback loops. Feedback loops work by sensing if a hormone in the body is too low or too high. The main orchestration of all of this starts with the hypothalamus gland in the brain, which sends signals to the pituitary gland (called the "master gland"). Then, the pituitary gland communicates with the other main glands in the body which are responsible for the production of all the major hormones: cortisol, estrogen, progesterone, thyroid hormones and many others. It may all seem complex, but all you need is the basic idea of how the body strives for balance, the overall role of your hormones, and how to go about balancing them for optimal health.

I will start this chapter by explaining the basic interactions of the two female sex hormones (estrogen and progesterone), with the stress hormone cortisol. These three basic hormones will be mentioned in each chapter and serve as a foundation to your mood, weight and overall health.

1

Additionally this book will cover . . .

Chapter 1—How the basic stress-induced hormonal shift affects the mind and body.

Chapter 2—How this hormonal shift worsens with age, causes menopausal symptoms, and for some may require the use of synthetic hormones (HRT) to ease these symptoms.

Chapter 3 (revised) —How this hormonal shift impacts health causing stubborn weight gain and a slowed metabolism making more specific ketogenic diets and glandular protocols necessary.

Chapter 4—How this hormonal shift negatively impacts the thyroid gland causing thyroid symptoms resulting in the increased use of thyroid medication.

Chapter 5—How this hormonal shift causes PMS and menstrual dysfunctions that result in an increased use of the Birth Control Pill (BCP).

Chapter 6—How this hormonal shift negatively impacts mood and mental health resulting in an increased use of strong psychotropic medications.

Chapter 7—How this hormonal shift affects the speed of the body's aging process and the exploration of the hormone, HGH, to reverse this.

Chapter 8—Simple, safe and fast solutions to get rid of all symptoms by "Shifting" hormones back to where they should be by using the natural hormone balancing protocol!

Chapter 9 (new addition)—How this hormonal shift negatively impacts hair growth cycles causing hair loss and thinning over time.

The Delicate Balance of Estrogen, Progesterone and Cortisol

Our bodies need the stress hormone, cortisol, to buffer us from stress, even if it is sometimes touted in the media as a "fat-promoting" hormone. We also need adequate levels of estrogen and progesterone for optimal health and childbearing. Problems begin to arise when these basic sex and stress hormones get out of balance. Therefore, let us take a closer look at them. When it comes to weight problems, moodiness, and risk for health issues or disease; estrogen is the "bad guy" when it is out of balance with progesterone. This female sex hormone is responsible for fat and fluid retention and is also associated with certain neuro-chemicals that will cause you to feel more anxious and depressed, or at the very least, irritable with mood swings. On the other hand, progesterone—the other major female sex hormone— is considered the "good guy" when it comes to weight, mood, and overall health. Progesterone is also associated with the production of certain neuro-chemicals that soothe and relax the body and aid in sleep. Progesterone is also a fat burner and a diuretic—which helps to control weight and blood pressure—and therefore, it is needed to balance out estrogen. This hormone keeps the body healthy and your symptoms at bay.

Let us now look at a more detailed list of each of these hormone's roles before we discuss the issues that arise when they become imbalanced.

Estrogen will:

- Promote formation of female secondary sex characteristics

- Stimulate endometrial growth, breast tissue proliferation (growth) and cause the uterine lining to grow monthly

- Increase vaginal lubrication, thicken the vaginal walls

- Maintain vessels and skin (softness, thickness)

- Reduce bone re-absorption (loss), increase bone formation

- Increase platelet adhesiveness

- Increase HDL and triglycerides; decrease LDL fat deposition

- Cause salt (sodium) and water retention

- Reduce bowel motility (increase constipation)

- Increase cholesterol in bile

- Support hormone-sensitive breast cancers

Progesterone will:

- Play a role in regulating the menstrual cycle to ensure monthly periods

- Prepare the body for pregnancy; developing the lining of the uterus (endometrium) until menstruation or fertilization

- Bring on menstruation when levels drop as the uterine lining begins to break down

- Aid in avoiding symptoms of PMS and menopause by balancing out estrogen

- Aid the body in fat-burning and act as a natural diuretic to keep blood pressure stabilized

- Have a protective effect against breast cancers by balancing out estrogen

- Keep androgens (male-acting hormones) in check; adequate progesterone will prevent the conversion of testosterone to DHT (dihydrotestosterone—a bad form of testosterone) helping to prevent acne, skin oiliness, excess facial and body hair, and thinning of the hair on the head

We need both of these essential sex hormones, but keeping them in balance is necessary for our health, mood and proper weight management. A good metaphor to explain the "excitatory" role of estrogen and the "inhibitory" role of progesterone is the following: when the "parent" (progesterone) is around, the "teenager" (estrogen) behaves, but in the absence or lacking of the "parent" (progesterone), the "teenager" (estrogen) gets into trouble. Scientifically, this means that progesterone keeps estrogen in balance by preventing it from stimulating the receptor sites of the cells in an excitatory way, which if left unchecked, could cause too much cell growth and division. This can lead to problems such as fibrocystic breasts (or eventually breast cancer if other factors are present), endometriosis (too much buildup of tissue on the ovaries or uterus), or even excessively heavy periods due to too much build up of the lining of the uterus. These are all common examples of more serious health issues that can occur when estrogen's proliferation role is out of control along with our issues with PMS, mood, weight and energy.

Nature intended for progesterone and estrogen to be in balance and for each to play their role as directed by the pituitary gland. In this naturally balanced state, the body functions properly and ovulation (the release of a mature egg from the ovary) occurs with a menstrual cycle on time and with ease. Later on, menopause follows without uncomfortable symptoms. As a matter of fact, there are developed but less stressed-filled countries in other parts of the world, such as in South America, Europe and Asia, where they do not even have words for PMS and menopause as they do not suffer from the symptoms in the way that American women do. So, what is responsible for causing the major imbalance between estrogen and progesterone, and what is causing a host of other symptoms in American women? The answer is stress, or more specifically, the need for the increased production of the stress hormone, cortisol.

Stress plays the primary and most influential role in creating hormonal imbalances. Occasional stress that triggers an adrenaline release from the adrenal gland, like seeing a dangerous animal in the wild and running from it to safety, does not have long-term detrimental effects. The body was meant to deal with life-threatening stress from time to time. However, in our postmodern society, we are under constant or chronic stress, which the body is not programmed to handle as well. Because of this, we end up in a chronic state of "fight-or-flight," where the body puts a constant demand on the adrenal gland to produce cortisol in order to buffer us from stress. If the adrenal gland did not function in this way, we could literally die when a life-threatening situation occurred.

The adrenal gland must prepare the body by speeding up the heart-rate, releasing adrenaline, slowing digestion, and increasing sugar and insulin production. Our bodies were not made to adapt to this constant drain on our cortisol levels, and over time, the adrenal gland runs out of the "reserves" needed to manufacture cortisol. This starts the process of what can be called "adrenal fatigue," where the gland produces high levels of cortisol for extended periods of time. This ultimately can lead to "adrenal exhaustion." Adrenal exhaustion occurs when cortisol levels become overly depleted and the potential for other serious diseases can occur. This high demand for cortisol results in the body's need to steal "building blocks" so that it can make more of these reserves.

Can you guess what the body uses when it needs "building blocks" to produce more cortisol? It converts the very hormone that we need to keep us happy and in balance—progesterone—the "good guy." This is because progesterone is molecularly very close to cortisol, and therefore is easy for the body to convert. This back-up and for "emergency use only" plan is now a daily happening for American women of all ages.

This is, of course, an oversimplification of the complex pathway that hormones go through in order to convert into one another, but this scenario—from progesterone to cortisol—is the most important to understand. This is why stress is the foundation of the basic hormone shift leading to all hormonal imbalances and subsequent symptoms. Without delving into the detailed process, it is also important to know that other sex hormones (like estrogen and testosterone) can also be depleted by the body's constant demand for cortisol over a longer period of time.

The result of the body's unrelenting demand for cortisol causes us to have low progesterone, leaving us in a position of having too much estrogen in relation to progesterone (see Figure 1-1). This state is accompanied by any of the varying symptoms associated with premenstrual syndrome, peri- menopause, and menopause (see questionnaire at the end of this chapter to note symptoms). The degree of your imbalance will determine the amount and severity of your symptoms.

Figure 1-1
Imbalances in Female Hormone

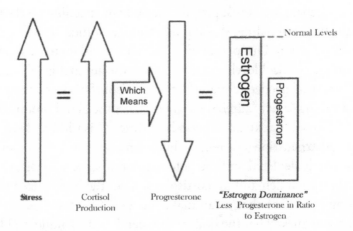

| Stress | Cortisol Production | Progesterone | "Estrogen Dominance" Less Progesterone in Ratio to Estrogen |

Too much estrogen in relation to progesterone is known as "estrogen dominance," a term coined by Dr. John Lee, an influential and integrative hormone researcher, whom is considered a pioneer in progesterone therapy. Most significantly, it has been shown by Dr. Lee's work, as well as others, that incidences of female-related cancers, including breast cancer and ovarian cancer, can increase with extreme *"estrogen dominance."* I quote some of Dr. Lee's work in a few of the applicable chapters.

Details on How Sex Hormones are Made and Depleted

There are three main estrogens in the body: estradiol, estrone, and estriol. Estradiol is the strongest, most abundant, and most active form of estrogen which I will be referring to most frequently. But, just for your understanding, there are two others—one of which is important after menopause, called estrone. Estrone is a weaker estrogen, made by the ovaries and fat tissue, and can be used as a "stored" estrogen so that estradiol can be made out of it later. Estriol, the third estrogen I will mention, is made by the placenta during pregnancy and is tested as a gauge for fetal distress. Levels of estriol do not change much after menopause and are the same in men as well.

The body has two ways, or pathways, of producing estrogen. Estradiol is made from testosterone and estrone is produced from androstenedione—both of which are made from a hormone called DHEA. DHEA (dehydroepiandrosterone) is a versatile steroidal hormone made by the adrenal gland and the gonads (in females this is our ovaries). It is created from pregnenolone, a master hormone made in the body from cholesterol (depicted in Figure 1-2). This process then starts the conversions of hormones to others as needed by the body.

This concept is important, because when long-term stress occurs and progesterone is depleted through its conversion to cortisol, levels of DHEA can also become depleted as well. I refer to this as "second-level" depletion (see Figure 1-3).

Figure 1-2
Simplified Hormone "Breakdown" Pathways

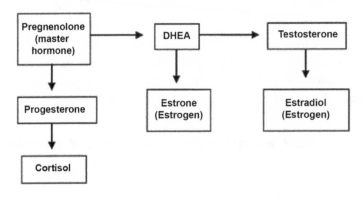

"Second-level" depletion only happens after long-term periods of stress (any type—physical or mental/emotional) and months or years of adrenal fatigue. It will likely result in true adrenal exhaustion, which reveals itself as low levels of cortisol on a lab test. In this case, DHEA levels become reduced as well, followed by falling estrogen and testosterone levels.

Figure 1-3
"Second Level" Hormone Depletion

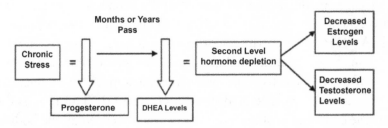

If you were to do a saliva test of estrogen, progesterone, cortisol and DHEA to see if you were hormonally imbalanced, the initial stage of this imbalance would show low progesterone levels, moderately to slightly elevated estrogen levels in conjunction with high cortisol levels (cortisol being made from progesterone, creating "estrogen dominance"), and adequate DHEA levels. This is a classic common sex and stress hormonal imbalance and would be classified as adrenal fatigue. The later stage of this hormonal imbalance would show very low progesterone levels, a slight to moderate decline in estrogen levels ("estrogen dominance" is still the case), low cortisol levels, and at this point a slight to moderate decrease in DHEA levels. This stage would be classified as adrenal *exhaustion.*

This "second-level" of depletion will then hinder the production of estrogen and testosterone and certain symptoms can appear; such as low libido, lack of motivation, vaginal dryness, thinning vaginal walls (causing painful intercourse), and bone loss. You will know if you are on your way to this type of scenario as you will have hot flashes and night sweats, which is simply the hypothalamus reacting to your falling estrogen levels in the bloodstream. Interestingly though, hot flashes and night sweats are always triggered by blood sugar falling. The falling estrogen levels in the bloodstream then affect the regularity of your menstrual cycle and can cause heavy periods (addressed more in Chapter 5). This is due to the existence of enough estrogen to stimulate the growth of the uterine lining but not enough estrogen to stimulate ovulation. This is called an "annovulatory cycle" (no ovulation), which results in the lack of production of progesterone at the spot where the egg is released. This progesterone is needed to halt the action of estrogen in building a heavy uterine lining. Later, when estrogen gets even lower (closer to menopause), then periods can be missed as there is not enough estrogen production for ovulation and not enough estrogen to build the uterine lining. This does not happen overnight but after many years of chronic stress (physical, mental and/ or emotional). This is rare in younger women (unless under extreme long-term stress) but it can become more common as you age. This type of situation can often be remedied without adding estrogen and testosterone, but rather by addressing the adrenal fatigue/exhaustion and by supplementing with DHEA and progesterone (explained in detail in Chapter 8).

Keep in mind that *most women* have the condition of "estrogen dominance" even when their estrogen drops as they age and they near menopause. This is because progesterone bottoms out and leaves you "estrogen dominant" even if your estrogen is being reduced. It is all about ratios and balance. The key, which is discussed throughout this book, is lowering stress and increasing progesterone; resulting in a balancing and stabilizing effect on your estrogen levels.

It is very important to note that estrogen is rarely ever low in the body; sometimes, after menopause it may be, due simply to the fact that progesterone levels were so low for so long because of stress or the long- term unnecessary use of a synthetic estrogen. Therefore, estrogen levels decrease as well because the body actually slows its production of it in order to achieve some sort of balance. If progesterone is increased, the body will adapt to these levels rising and begin to start to produce natural estrogen again.

If estrogen ever seems to be low in a younger (pre-menopausal) woman, it is usually not truly low levels of estrogen but just a deactivation of the estrogen receptor sites (they become less sensitive to circulating estrogen). This can happen when progesterone levels have been low over an extended period of time and can easily be corrected when progesterone levels are raised. It is also important to understand that the basic imbalance of estrogen and progesterone, resulting in "estrogen dominance," tends to worsen with time as a woman gets closer to menopause. Oftentimes, the one week of PMS-related symptoms grows into three weeks of feeling awful. The end result being one week each month where you actually feel good! This is the start of what women dread about menopause, and it makes it even harder to manage mood, weight, and sleep; or to even have the energy to try!

When There is an Abrupt Change in Hormones

When a total hysterectomy (ovaries removed as well) is performed—basically, a surgical menopause—it is usually because of problems related to "estrogen dominance;" such as precancerous cells, endometriosis, uterine fibroids, or cysts. These issues are all caused by estrogen overreacting on the body's tissues. After a hysterectomy, the body will still exhibit a host of symptoms because it has now abruptly lost a main supplier of estrogen (estradiol). Now, the body has to learn to adapt to a new source of estrogen, called estrone, which is produced in the skin and fat cells and even parts of the brain when progesterone levels are adequate. In the case when a hysterectomy is needed, you would have been drastically low in progesterone to begin with, or you would not have had the above- mentioned symptoms and needed the hysterectomy. So, now you will be deficient in progesterone *and* natural estrogen! At this point, you are in dire need of progesterone as it will immediately ease most of your pre-existing symptoms and it will allow the body to start to want to balance out. This addition of progesterone will stimulate the body to start to produce natural estrogen, estrone, on its own from the body's fat stores. Estrone is the chief estrogen in women after menopause and should provide an adequate amount of estrogen long term if progesterone is at optimum levels. The only reason that estrone levels do not adequately rise is because progesterone levels are too low for a prolonged period of time. Because of this, the body attempts to maintain homeostasis (balance); and therefore, it will forego the production of estrone until progesterone levels increase. This is when hormone replacement therapy (synthetic or bio-identical) or the birth control pill is often used to attempt to balance female hormones (This will be discussed in Chapter 2 and Chapter 5).

Additional Key Hormones Affecting a Woman's Health

Let us start with the two main hormones that play an important role in orchestrating a woman's monthly cycle and her ability to conceive, follicle- stimulating hormone (FSH) and luteinizing hormone (LH). They will be mentioned again in Chapter 2 and Chapter 5 of the book. These hormones are both produced by the pituitary gland when signaled to do so by the hypothalamus gland. Their names denote the phase in which they are most active. FSH is most active in the first fourteen days of a woman's twenty- eight day cycle called the "follicular" phase where it attaches to receptors on the follicles stimulating their growth and also causes the release of estrogen. This phase then culminates in mid-cycle ovulation (releasing of the egg to be fertilized) as LH surges starting the second half of the menstrual cycle called the "luteal" phase. LH also aids in the development of the corpus luteum (the spot where the follicle is released from) to allow it to produce progesterone. When the corpus luteum disintegrates, a new twenty- eight day cycle begins. It is important to note that FSH and LH act synergistically in reproduction.

Later in life, as a woman approaches menopause, she will often deal with stubborn excess weight that cannot be lost with traditional diet and exercise (even when adhered to strictly). Weight loss needs to be addressed in its own separate chapter because many hormonal imbalances will cause weight gain and all the other PMS and menopausal symptoms. I had addressed this issue in Chapter 3 in the first edition of my book by discussing my past success with using the homeopathic hormone hCG (human chorionic gonadotropin) to overcome this weight loss barrier. Now that this hormone is off the market in the safe homeopathic form, I will discuss in this revised chapter, how glandular therapies can be used instead for the same effect but with lasting results. Glandular therapies involve utilizing glands, organs or tissue from healthy animals to improve the function of the same glands/organs in the patient or client. Glandular tissue extracts come in pill form or homeopathic form for all the major glands of the body such as the hypothalamus, pituitary, adrenal, ovarian as well as the most widely used gland today, the thyroid gland. I will discuss how this gentle glandular therapy can be safe, easy to use and aid in resetting the hypothalamus' ability to orchestrate the entire hormone cascade. This process will aid in resetting the metabolism when combined with a specific low calorie diet plan that brings the body into a healthy state of ketosis. This calming state of ketosis, which will be explained, will also raise progesterone and aid in stabilizing blood sugar and corisol levels having a positive impact on the adrenal gland.

Now that you understand how important it is to raise progesterone levels that have been drained in order to make cortisol due to excessive stress, you will come to see how beneficial a initial temporary, ketogenic state is along with some glandular support to restoring this balance for any woman with a hormonal imbalance. This concept will become clearer in Chapter 3 when I explain the hormonal benefits that my clients are experiencing while using our specific ketogenic diet with a homeopathic glandular blend for even the most stubborn weight pre, peri, or post menopause.

In Chapter 4, I will touch on the thyroid hormones, T3 and T4, which are produced by the thyroid gland and peripheral tissues of the body. They are made from the amino acid, tyrosine. It is well known that thyroid hormones are responsible for regulating many aspects of our metabolism. The ratio of T4 to T3 in the blood is 20 to 1, but T3 is important and is three to four times more active than T4. The thyroid's working process begins in the brain. The hypothalamus tells the pituitary gland to produce thyroid-stimulating hormone (TSH).

TSH in turn stimulates the thyroid gland to produce more T4 to be made into T3 when blood levels of these hormones are low. If there are adequate amounts of T3 and T4 in the blood and the feedback system is working correctly, you should have normal TSH levels on a blood test. However, "estrogen dominance" and adrenal fatigue, brought on by stress, will negatively affect thyroid function. There is also the concern that the standard thyroid tests, which are used as a basis for medication prescription, are not completely accurate or applicable anymore. This controversy will be discussed in Chapter 4.

Insulin is a key hormone in the body that controls blood sugar. It is directly affected by stress and the release of cortisol in the body. When we are under stress, cortisol is released into the bloodstream as well as sugar to help us "flee" the danger, and this is always followed by the release of insulin in order to aid in lowering blood sugar. It is important to note that it is not just what we eat (sugar, alcohol, caffeine) that will cause a rise in blood sugar, followed by a rise in insulin. When we are stressed at work or thinking stressful thoughts throughout our day (self hatred, insecurity, fear, etc.), a constant release of cortisol will result in a release of blood sugar followed by insulin, which eventually leads to a condition called "insulin resistance." We think of "insulin resistance" as the precursor for diabetes, which is true, but it can cause stubborn issues with your weight and mood swings (depression/ anxiety) as well. This is further discussed in Chapter 3 and Chapter

The hormone imbalance of "estrogen dominance" will exacerbate "insulin resistance" just as "insulin resistance" will exacerbate "estrogen dominance." It is a vicious cycle. Progesterone tends to have a buffering effect on blood sugar and positively affects your mood, weight, and sleep. When you do not get enough sleep, or when you go to bed and just cannot sleep, you become more "insulin resistant" and your brain's neuro-chemicals can easily become imbalanced, which parallels your hormone imbalance. This will also be discussed in Chapter 6. A part of this process is the lowering of a hormone called melatonin. Melatonin is essential for sleep and its depletion can lead to insomnia. Melatonin regulates the sleep cycle so its production is easily affected by lightness and darkness. It is produced from the amino acid, tryptophan, and it is secreted mostly through the spinal fluid. I will discuss why this occurs in Chapter 6, as well as how it affects mood.

In Chapter 7, I will discuss Human Growth Hormone (HGH) in relation to aging and how it can be used to slow this process. HGH is produced by somatotropic cells in the anterior pituitary gland located deep within the brain. It is the most abundant hormone produced from this gland because over forty percent of the cells in the pituitary gland are somatotropic cells. Sometimes, called the "master hormone," its role is to affect every cell in a child's body as they grow. In adults, it will aid in regenerating, repairing, and replicating cells. Our stressful lives as adults will cause hormonal imbalances that speed the aging process. In order to curb the effects of stress on the body, overall stress needs to be reduced, sex and stress hormones need to be balanced and innovative new ways to slow aging (like the use of HGH) can make dramatic changes.

The Importance of Controlling Stress

What can we do to control our stress in order to help avoid adrenal fatigue and eventually adrenal exhaustion? We need to evaluate our lifestyle and rid ourselves of as much stress as we can. While it is true that we create a lot of our own stress, it also comes in the form of noise, bright city lights, constantly ringing cell phones, commitments, careers, school, children, taxes, and so on; all of which over-stimulate our systems. As women, naturally, we are multi-taskers, which is stressful in and of itself and inhibits us from being able to "shut off our brains" at the end of the day.

Keep in mind that stress can be physical, mental, emotional, and even spiritual. In case you are unsure about your stress level, take a look at the following types of stress and determine for yourself if you are affected by them:

Physical Issues: Lack of sleep, intense exercise, blood sugar fluctuations from food or stressful thoughts, pain, toxins in the body, artificial light, digestive weaknesses, yeasts/parasites in the body, chronic health conditions, electromagnetic fields (EMF's) in your environment, poor air quality.

Mental Issues: Any complex problem that you cannot solve, repetitive thoughts from the past, financial planning/concerns, interpersonal issues/interactions, complex planning of future events, job or scholastic responsibilities.

Emotional Issues (conscious and subconscious): Unresolved childhood traumas, lack of love or nurturing, unprocessed negative emotions stored in the body (such as anger or bitterness toward parents or an ex spouse), self-limiting beliefs, self-esteem issues, lack of authenticity in your life, lack of a spiritual connection.

These are all common chronic stress issues that can be more of a challenge when met with temporary stressful events like moving to a new home, starting a new job, having a child, getting married, and so on.

I doubt that you will be able to quit your job, leave your husband, or drop your kids off at a *never- ending* sleep-over camp, so I imagine that you are experiencing some type of stress that is throwing your body out of whack. This is where, in Chapter 8, I can help you to understand how proper, safe supplementation with completely natural hormones can be very effective in helping you lead the full, fun, and stimulating life you deserve—free of uncomfortable symptoms related to hormonal imbalances.

Common Symptoms of Hormonal Imbalances Associated with PMS and Menopause

If you have any of the following symptoms, you most likely have a hormonal imbalance:

- Chronic Low Energy
- Constipation
- Depression/Anxiety
- Foggy Thinking
- Food Cravings
- Hair Loss
- Excess Facial or Body Hair Growth

- Lack of Libido
- Breast Tenderness
- Fibrocystic Breasts
- Fibroids
- Endometriosis
- Ovarian Pain/Cysts
- Mood Swings

- Headaches
- Hot Flashes/Night Sweats
- Insomnia
- Irregular Periods
- Heavy Periods
- Irritability
- Joint Pain/Inflammation

- PMS (combination of many symptoms listed lasting up to a full week before your period)
- Poor Memory
- Weight Gain/Fluid Retention (Bloating)
- Acne
- Melasma (dark patches on skin)

The body knows how to produce enough hormones in order for it to run properly; therefore, the balance between all of the varying types of hormones can be maintained under normal conditions. However, a chronic stressful lifestyle can upset this balance—resulting in a hormonal "Shift." The type and severity of your symptoms also slightly depends on your genetics. Genetically, this involves your total ovarian and adrenal capacity to produce hormones, as well as nutritional deficiencies, enzyme reserves, and inherited immune or digestive weaknesses. All of these combine and result in your specific mixture of symptoms. Rest assured, as we probably will never fully discover or understand these complexities, basic hormonal balance can be achieved once you understand the reasons for your imbalance.

Research and Experienced-Based Facts

The following is a summary of my health center's findings over the past years:

1. **Most women do need to supplement their hormones if they display symptoms of hormone-related imbalances.**

Let us face it, if you felt great, looked great, and were sleeping great, you would not be reading this book. Unfortunately, most women who have PMS or menopausal symptoms are "estrogen dominant," which means they have low levels of progesterone in relation to estrogen. Based on research, estrogen levels themselves are usually not the problem. "Estrogen dominance" can cause all of the hormone-related symptoms, including (but not limited to) PMS, hot flashes, irritability, headaches, depression, anxiety, weight gain, bloating, low energy, low motivation and willpower. Assuming you are "estrogen dominant," it will be virtually impossible for you to look and feel your best throughout every stage of your life without proper supplementation to increase your levels of progesterone. A completely natural and highly absorbable source will be described in great detail in Chapter 8 of this book.

2. Stopping the conversion of progesterone to cortisol is necessary to maintain long-term hormonal balance.

We know that increased stress causes an increase in the body's need to produce cortisol because it buffers us from this stress. Over a long period of chronic stress, the body runs out of the reserves to make cortisol, which leads to what we call adrenal fatigue. The body then needs to convert or steal progesterone to use as building blocks in order to manufacture the much-needed cortisol. This leaves a woman in a state of imbalance, which is reflected by her levels of progesterone and cortisol on lab tests.

Only when this stress response is addressed, will a woman's supplemented progesterone remain at the proper levels to allow her to rebalance and maintain that balance. It is rare for doctors to address this issue, but addressing adrenal fatigue/exhaustion is the key to getting hormones truly balanced long term. In addition to important lifestyle modifications, natural methods—including homeopathy and hormone balancing creams—can calm the adrenal gland when you are under stress so that the body does not need to exhaust your supply of progesterone. This will be discussed later in this book.

3. Natural hormone replacement does not cause the side effects or unnatural buildup that is often associated with synthetic hormones.

When a completely natural hormone solution is used, such as the progesterone based cream I use in my center, it works with the body to balance the hormones without side effects. Side effects are usually only seen with synthetic compounds, pharmaceutical drugs, or pharmaceutical compounded solutions—some of which are foreign to the body. Natural solutions support the entire endocrine system (which comprises the body's hormone-producing glands) in order to help diminish the "estrogen dominance" symptoms without the unpleasant side effects.

The body is often able to rebalance with a natural solution and will not overproduce any of the sex hormones. Also, there is no danger of a buildup in the fatty tissue. For this reason, it is usually unnecessary to test hormone levels with natural hormone replacement (see #6 below). More about the dangers of hormones building up in the body and other side effects with synthetic hormone supplementation is discussed in Chapter 2.

4. Any woman who is carrying around excess weight is affected by a hormonal imbalance.

While there are other contributing factors to weight gain and excess weight, such as "insulin resistance," hormonal imbalances are always playing a role as well. Insulin is a chief player in the body because it controls blood sugar levels, and it responds to what we eat as well as the stress that we feel. In women, elevated insulin levels almost always go hand-in-hand with seemingly high estrogen levels (meaning estrogen that is not being "balanced out" by progesterone). This, in conjunction with low progesterone levels (progesterone is a natural fat-burner and diuretic), makes it difficult to lose weight, which is even more difficult as a woman approaches her forties or gets closer to menopause. Women usually suspect that a hormonal imbalance is at play when they have difficulty losing weight. Fortunately, there is a completely natural way to address this weight problem that I use in my health center and you will learn more about it in Chapter 3.

5. Estrogen or testosterone supplementation is rarely necessary and can in fact, be dangerous.

Testosterone, the male sex hormone, is rarely shown to be low on a woman's saliva lab tests; and therefore, does not usually need to be supplemented. Furthermore, as I mentioned earlier, low levels of estrogen are also rarely ever the cause of the hormone-related symptoms we are discussing in this book. In my health center, I never suggest supplementing with testosterone or estrogen. From lab research, we know that when progesterone levels are where they should be, estrogen will also be at optimum levels because the body can easily produce estrogen to maintain a balance between the two (from fat or skin). Additionally, the issues that seem to be related to low testosterone (low sex drive and motivation) will balance as well, without the need to force the body in one direction by administering direct testosterone. There are a few exceptions, however, but this is also the most conservative approach and the method with which I choose to use. Of those mentioned so far, progesterone is the only supplemental hormone that has been studied long term (by Dr. Lee) and has been proven safe!

6. While saliva testing is more accurate than blood testing for hormone levels, it can be expensive and is usually not necessary if the course of treatment is completely natural.

The best way to test hormone levels is through saliva testing, which shows free hormones, not bound to proteins, available for use by the body. Blood tests typically show both, free and bound hormones (bound to proteins), so an accurate reading is not as easily determined. Because of the expense, I use saliva testing in my center only in extreme cases (such as cancer) or if a woman wishes to know her exact levels. When using a completely natural hormone solution, such as the supplements I use, blood or saliva testing is unnecessary. With natural solutions, there are no side effects or risks of toxicity or buildup. Also, keep in mind that the primary way you will know your hormones are balanced is when your hormone- related symptoms cease to be an issue for you. This is your body telling you that you are balanced! More on this topic will be discussed in Chapter 2.

8. Most general practitioners have little or no substantial education regarding hormone levels.

If you are wondering why your doctor brushes away your concerns regarding your hormones or is unfamiliar with the information I present in this book, it is important to know that it is not your doctor's fault. Like nutrition, medical students receive very few hours of training on sex hormones and learn most of the other information from pharmaceutical companies who are promoting oral contraceptives, synthetic hormone-replacement therapies, Viagra, pain medications, and antidepressants. All of these options simply mask symptoms and produce many side effects. Surgeries, such as hysterectomies and ablations (the removal of the inside of the uterine lining by use of a laser or high frequency electrical energy), are often performed unnecessarily due to a misunderstanding of a simple hormonal imbalance that can be corrected.

Of course, there are some medical doctors who have studied hormones in depth and offer prescriptions for compounded formulas called bio-identical therapy. While compounded bio-identical hormones are one step closer to a natural solution, the model of testing can be flawed. These types of hormones given are not proven safe for long-term usage. There is usually no work with adrenal fatigue/exhaustion, and some of the delivery systems used can result in a buildup of hormones in the fatty tissue; therefore, this is not the solution I recommend to my clients. Doctors also need to monitor hormone levels with saliva or blood testing yearly when using bio-identical hormone therapy. More about bio-identical hormone therapy can be found in Chapter 2.

The following symptom based questionnaire will aid you in seeing how out of balance your hormones are. This translates to how "estrogen dominant" you are. Typically, the more symptoms on this comprehensive list you suffer from, the greater your hormonal imbalance. There are always exceptions to this in that you may suffer from only a few symptoms on the list but they are severe in nature. An example may be painful, heavy periods with endometriosis. There are only 2-3 symptoms tied into this case but these indicate a fairly big imbalance in sex hormones.

Hormone Imbalance Questionnaire:

Circles "Y" (yes) for each symptoms that applies to you.

Hot Flashes	Y / N	Brittle nails	Y / N	Hypoglycemic tendencies	Y / N
Night Sweats	Y / N	Hair Loss	Y / N	Bloating after meals	Y / N

Irritability	Y / N	Acne	Y/N	Fibrocystic Breasts	Y / N
Depression	Y / N	Headaches	Y / N	Breast Tenderness	Y / N
Anxiety	Y / N	Vaginal Dryness	Y / N	Breast Cancer	Y / N
Mood Swings	Y / N	Lack of libido	Y / N	Uterine Fibroids	Y / N
Irregular Periods	Y / N	Insomnia	Y / N	Endometriosis	Y / N
Heavy Periods	Y / N	Yeast Infections	Y / N	Ovarian Pain	Y / N
Painful Periods	Y / N	Memory Loss	Y / N	Ovarian tumors or cysts	Y / N
Weight Gain	Y / N	Sweet or Salt Cravings	Y / N	PMS	Y / N

Answer the following two questions if you are postmenopausal (no period for one year either as a result of surgery or stage of life)

Did you begin menopause prior to the age of 55 yrs?	Y / N
Was your menopause surgically induced?	Y / N

Total "yes" answers: _____

If you answered "yes" fewer than two to three times, your hormone imbalance is considered **MILD**. Hormone therapy is optional. Consider reducing your stress levels to alleviate these symptoms.

If you answered "yes" more than three times but fewer than ten, your hormone imbalance is considered **MODERATE**. Consider safe and natural hormone balancing to rid yourself of these bothersome symptoms.

If you answered "yes" more than ten times, your hormone balance is considered **SEVERE**. Consider safe and natural hormone balancing to rid yourself of these symptoms as well as aid in preventing more serious health issues in the future.

If you would like to take a more detailed hormone assessment online, please go to bebalancedcenters.com and complete it there. A natural hormone balancing specialist will follow-up with you to go over your results.

Hopefully, you now understand the basics of the main female sex hormones and how they can dramatically influence your daily life. I have also addressed a few other key hormones that will affect your mood, weight and health. Chronic stress and its repercussions on the entire endocrine system is the core reason we manifest PMS and menopausal symptoms, gain weight and age rapidly.

Now that this foundation has been set, we can use this to further delve into how the hormone shift can cause imbalances in seven different areas with a discussion how natural hormone balancing can safely and quickly diminish all the PMS and menopausal symptoms caused by it. Final solutions that are natural, safe and effective will be presented in Chapter 8 with the hair loss/thinning solutions presented in the newly added Chapter 9.

CHAPTER 2

The Hormone Shift & Menopause

The Use of HRT to Treat Symptoms . . .

Why do women experience menopausal symptoms?
Why are so many women put on synthetic hormones?
Why is estrogen the hormone often prescribed?
Why does synthetic estrogen seem to work temporarily?
What are the dangers of excess estrogen?
What are the issues with synthetic and bio-identical hormone therapy?
Solution: Use natural hormone balancing to relieve menopausal symptoms Specifics on a natural hormone balancing solution (refer to Chapter 8)

Most women experience uncomfortable symptoms around the menopausal years because of a further shift in hormones. The timing of the onset of these symptoms can vary depending on stress levels. It is understood that stress causes the shift or imbalance of the female hormones, which culminates in the many symptoms around menopause. Now, the question is, "Why are women told that menopausal symptoms are caused by low estrogen levels when most hormonal symptoms are really caused by an imbalance of estrogen and progesterone?" This misconception is then exacerbated by administering extra estrogen, in either a synthetic or bio-identical form, in order to ease chronic symptoms.

Many women find themselves asking, "Do I have to either learn how to 'deal with' my menopausal symptoms on my own, or risk the dangerous side effects associated with synthetic hormone replacement therapy (HRT) prescribed by my doctor?" In my experience, the answer is, "No." There are natural ways to eradicate the symptoms of menopause quickly, effectively, and without dangerous side effects by replacing the correct hormone that is deficient with a non-synthetic source and by treating the main cause of its deficiency, which is an adrenal issue.

Menopause should not be a time of total discomfort. The symptoms that many American women experience during this stage of life are usually a result of a high-stress modern lifestyle, as stated in Chapter

In countries where women are not exposed to the same level of toxic chemicals, stressful lifestyles, and poor nutrition, they experience menopause as a natural transition; which is to be celebrated. When the time is right, should we not celebrate the freedom of no longer getting periods? A more recent trend is for menopausal symptoms to occur prematurely in American women because they are under severe stress for extended periods of time. However, they are really not in true menopause at all, they are just prematurely experiencing the annoying symptoms!

To be clear, I would like to define this menopausal phase of life. The definition of menopause that I choose to adopt is "the true cessation of ovarian function" as a woman approaches her mid-fifties. This should be natural and is expected. Nearing this point, the ovaries do not produce enough estrogen and this causes ovulation to slow. This inability to ovulate can cause heavy periods (discussed in detail in Chapter 5) or missed periods (discussed below) depending on the level of estrogen available at the time.

Menopause, defined by the medical community, is when a woman "has not had a period for close to a year" and at that point it can be assumed that she has probably stopped ovulating. I feel this is also another good definition for menopause, as a woman will obviously stop menstruating as she enters this phase. It coincides with my definition of menopause (true ovarian failure) as well. Naturally, this should usually occur in a woman's mid-fifties, but in America many women stop getting their periods in their forties and it can take up to a year for it to finally cease. By my definition, this woman is not truly in menopause as her ovaries still have working potential, but by the medical definition it can seem as if she is in true menopause. This can make things very confusing. This premature cessation of the menstrual cycle results from everyday stressors that literally drain progesterone levels, then DHEA levels, which in turn leads to lowered estrogen levels. When progesterone is drained and estrogen is lowered, there is often not enough estrogen to stimulate ovulation, even if there is enough estrogen remaining in order to build the uterine lining to induce a monthly period. Therefore, monthly menstrual cycles become irregular, and if you have experienced this, you sense that you are entering menopause. Eventually, the level of estrogen in the body drops so low that neither ovulation occurs nor does the lining build up, and you stop getting your period for twelve months straight. Usually, this transition starts prematurely but by the time you have gone a full twelve months with no period, you feel as if it is safe to say that you are in menopause.

How do you know if you are truly in menopause? A common test used by many doctors is the FSH (follicle-stimulating hormone) test. FSH rises and remains consistently high when the pituitary gland senses that ovulation has ceased due to truly low estrogen. This test is often given to women who seem to be experiencing fertility problems, but it can be used to confirm that menopause is near or presently occurring.

Do you ever wonder where the phrase peri-menopause comes from? It describes the phase between irregular menstrual cycles and true menopause (the cessation of ovarian function). However, the term peri-menopause is relatively new. It was only coined to address this difficult period of life of on-again, off-again periods, which are a direct result of our stressful lifestyle. This shift in hormones now has its own name dictating a phase of the unknown, "Will I get my period this month or not?"

This new phase is occurring because progesterone levels are left too low for too long and the estrogen that remains will have reduced effectiveness. This can happen even before DHEA levels drop and your actual estrogen levels drop, caused by what I call "second-level" depletion—as mentioned in Chapter 1. According to Dr. Lee (2004), in *What Your Doctor Did Not Tell You About Menopause,* progesterone aids in estrogen's effectiveness by making estrogen receptors more sensitive (p. 286). This loss of estrogen's effectiveness should not be confused with a true "lack of estrogen," and can occur in women in their late thirties and early forties bringing on these nasty menopausal symptoms at this pre-mature age. This is one of the reasons that hot flashes can start years before a woman should reach true menopause. Fortunately, in this case, I have observed that progesterone supplementation is a way to quickly relieve these symptoms. By keeping stress levels low and progesterone levels up, the transition into menopause can be much smoother, and peri-menopause can cease to be a concern. Peri-menopause and its affects could be so minimal that it would not even warrant its own term! Whatever the case may be, I do not think women care what phase they are in as long as it does not slow them down and cause an array of symptoms. Don't you agree? A symptom-free, on-the-go life can be achieved if stress levels are managed and normal levels of progesterone are maintained, which in turn helps to maintain healthy estrogen levels, even with age.

Treating Menopausal Symptoms Medically

The medical community seems to be addressing the issue of menopausal symptoms by comparison of risks versus benefits. Women are instructed to talk to their doctor about the symptoms they are experiencing during menopause or peri -menopause, and if certain symptoms become unbearable, then and only then, the doctor will recommend some form of synthetic hormonal replacement therapy (HRT).

Synthetic HRT is no longer the most immediate recommendation for women dealing with hormonal imbalance symptoms. The 2002 Women' s Initiative Study, involving 161,808 women, had to be cut short because of the endangerment of the health of the participants. It started in 1991 and was to last fifteen years. The National Heart, Lung, and Blood Institute (NHLBI) of the National Institutes of Health (NIH) stopped the trial use of the estrogen-plus-progestin a few years early because of the resulting increased risk of breast cancer in otherwise healthy menopausal women. This combination hormonal treatment was also found to increase the risk of strokes, pulmonary embolisms, and heart disease.

However, HRT is still prescribed commonly in extreme cases, such as when a woman's quality of life has deteriorated enough that she is willing to take that risk. It is truly a shame that a woman feels she must choose between a symptom-free life now—with the potential for a deadly disease later—or avoid HRT and simply live with her menopausal symptoms.

In working with the female clients at my center, I have repeatedly witnessed almost every menopausal symptom being eradicated with natural hormonal balancing. The specifics of how estrogen becomes imbalanced with progesterone were mentioned in Chapter 1 and a specific natural solution is later mentioned in Chapter 8.

You may ask, "Why don't doctors tell us that we can safely and naturally eradicate our uncomfortable symptoms?" It is because most doctors are not trained extensively in sex hormone and stress hormone interactions. Most of the information doctors receive comes from drug companies, which are, for lack of better words, pushing the birth control pill or synthetic hormone "solutions." These synthetic methods do work to relieve some major symptoms in most cases, but the mechanism through which they work is not the safest. This is evident to those who truly have a better understanding of how hormones interact in the body. Furthermore, we have to ask ourselves, "Can synthetic hormones really be a viable option for long-term symptom management when they have been directly linked to be the potential cause for deadly disease?" It would be beneficial if the medical community were more versed in this topic so that they could appropriately guide women through menopause. Currently, their recommended available options are synthetic hormones (HRT), complacency/symptom tolerance, or eventually major surgery.

So, why are so many women still taking synthetic hormones despite the side effects and risks? It is probably because they do not know that there is a fast, safe, effective, and natural alternative in "natural hormone balancing." Taking drugs is probably not anyone's first choice, but women often do so because they think they have no other way to deal with their extreme and persistent hormone-related symptoms. Furthermore, most people do not know that even though the drug therapies are approved by the FDA, only about ten percent of drugs have double-blind studies performed on them. A double blind study is one that protects the outcome from both biased results and placebo effects.

That being said, as many as ten percent of natural professional products that are sold through clinicians (not in health food stores) have had double- blind studies. Therefore, with that information, the assumption that all pharmaceuticals are studied more in-depth than natural supplementation is false. After the results of the *Women's Initiative Study* were made public, many doctors thought twice before prescribing synthetic HRT. The reason why doctors may still dispense synthetic HRT is because some women complain of horrible hot flashes and the doctors do not really have any other options to offer.

Estrogen-the Wrong Hormone Prescribed with HRT

Estrogen is the hormone most often thought to be deficient in menopausal women and peri-menopausal women leading to all the symptoms experienced. Hopefully now you understand the adrenal issues leading to low progesterone which are really the cause of the dreaded issues with mood, sleep, stubborn weight and the female cycle that occur around menopause or even peri-menopause. Due to the medical community not being well versed in this fact, estrogen is often prescribed in order to eradicate these symptoms as well symptoms of like hot flashes and night sweats. Interestingly enough, blood and saliva tests are always more likely to show much lower progesterone levels than estrogen levels even in a postmenopausal woman. Many doctors, however, still prescribe an estrogen patch or another synthetic estrogen, like Premarin, to a woman who complains about these symptoms. One simple reason this is done is because it will work in most cases to stop symptoms of low estrogen, such as hot flashes/night sweats, low libido, vaginal dryness, painful intercourse from thinning vaginal walls and overall bone loss. The problem is that a woman in this situation is not protected from female-related cancers and will be much more likely to gain weight around the midsection, feel irritable and have insomnia due to the extra estrogen.

The truly deficient hormone, progesterone, was not originally prescribed with the estrogen. However, it is now being given in a synthetic form, in combination with estrogen, if a woman still has a uterus. The idea for this is to protect against certain female-related cancers. This is important because estrogen alone acts on the cells' receptors in the breast, ovaries, and uterus in an excitatory or stimulatory way. A common example is Prempro, which is a synthetic blend of estrogen and progestin (synthetic progesterone). The use of estrogen in a synthetic form, when a woman is deficient in natural progesterone will then cause her imbalance of estrogen to progesterone to become even more imbalanced, and her long- term health could be jeopardized. The alternative of adding in synthetic progesterone (progestin) still offers no protection against breast cancer and will contribute to midsection weight gain and fluid retention. Please note, should you be prescribed an oral form of progesterone (which is micronized), this delivery system is quite inefficient (whether natural or synthetic) because most of it is unavailable to the body. It needs to travel through the digestive system, which in a stressed person, does not work efficiently. Massive doses are usually required in order to increase one's progesterone level and are often prescribed with ineffective outcomes.

In Chapter 5, you can read more on the ways that synthetic forms of progesterone will actually cause additional problems. This will be discussed in reference to the birth control pill (BCP). What you are not told, is that when using estrogen combined with progestin, you are technically still high in estrogen; therefore, what you really need in this situation is natural progesterone.

It is rare for a saliva test to reveal low estrogen levels before menopause. If the hormone tests do indicate low levels of estrogen at this time, it is often not a true deficit. This is because the adrenal gland, as well as the gonads (ovaries), produce both progesterone and estrogen. However, estrogen is unique in that it can easily be made by the fat and skin cells, as well as by parts of the brain in the form of estrone—a weaker stored form of estrogen. It is safe to say that most women have the capacity to be fairly "well stocked," in estrogen when compared with progesterone. When the ovaries no longer produce adequate estrogen, or if they are removed, other sources of estrogen should take over.

However, if you are premenopausal and happen to have extremely low progesterone, the body will try to compensate for this by stopping estrogen production in order to allow the progesterone levels to "catch up." Oftentimes, this balance is rarely achieved because stress keeps your progesterone levels low. In this scenario, you start to experience a host of other symptoms in addition to your original PMS symptoms, which you may have had for years due to "estrogen dominance." These symptoms start with estrogen "falling" which is often shown by hot flashes/night sweats and can progress into vaginal dryness and low libido. These are symptoms that a younger woman would typically not display. As mentioned, I have seen repeatedly, from saliva lab tests, that if a woman is administered a high quality progesterone (see Chapter 8), along with remedying her adrenal issues, her body will eventually start producing estrogen on its own through the ovaries (pre-menopausal) or through the fat stores (post menopausal). Some symptoms, such as low libido, may take longer to correct in these cases based on my observation.

Using Topical Estrogen for Extreme Cases

There are many women who cannot wait to alleviate their symptoms, such as vaginal dryness, because they are so severe. In these cases, the use of localized estrogen for a short period of time is the best available option. This will ease symptoms while the body starts to make natural estrogen on its own again. It is best to keep this estrogen localized to the vaginal tissue only. There is no proof, of course, that this estrogen stays localized, but this is the best alternative I have seen so far for this issue. Estriol (in its more natural form) of all three estrogens, tends to work best for vaginal tissue if your doctor can prescribe that for you. Unfortunately, a large pharmaceutical company has made this hormone almost impossible to obtain because it competes with their synthetic estrogen products. Believe it or not, this is even applicable for a compounding pharmacist, and therefore it may be some time before this is available to the public. Also, note that giving synthetic estrogen in the form of the patch—if a woman chooses to do so temporarily—will be better if it is used simultaneously with natural progesterone, in order to truly help protect her against female - related cancers (Lee, 1996, p. 324). This estrogen-patch alternative also seems to be less dangerous than the synthetic estrogen found in the BCP or oral estrogens, because it will bypass the liver process and reduce the risk of liver function alteration. This is not my first recommendation, but it can be used in extreme cases—in low doses and for short periods of time—with of course, some natural progesterone to balance it. I recommend this only after addressing adrenal fatigue/exhaustion and supplement progesterone to "reawaken" the body's estrogen production.

Long-term Use of Synthetic Hormones Will Suppress Natural Hormone Production

An important point to address with synthetic HRT, in the form of estrogen therapy, is that long-term use of this synthetic hormone will cause natural estrogen production to slow down or shut down altogether. There are many women who have been controlling their "estrogen dominance" symptoms with synthetic hormones like the BCP or HRT. A pattern I see is that when a woman's estrogen level is suppressed for so long, estrogen can take many months to rise to normal levels after cessation of the BCP or HRT is stopped. This will even be the case when natural progesterone therapy is introduced. This occurs because of years of abuse of synthetic hormones that have suppressed natural hormone production. Of course, synthetic hormones do suppress many undesirable symptoms like hot flashes (in an older woman) and can regulate a menstrual cycle (in a younger woman). However, these women are still plagued with other symptoms, and problems with gaining weight will eventually arise. They are also at a greater risk for developing female-related cancers, and their production of needed estrogen will not rebalance as quickly even with the use of a good, topical progesterone cream. For years, their bodies have not produced estrogen on their own because of the high levels of synthetic estrogen. The feedback system used to keep the body in balance may have been altered, and now the body has to be retrained. Balance can and will happen, but sadly, it will take much longer in these cases. Typically, this is a case when a woman used topical estrogen cream for the vaginal area, or the estrogen patch spoke of in the previous section.

How Safe Are the More Natural Bio-Identical Hormones?

Bio-identical hormones are more natural to the body than synthetic hormones. However, they are still altered chemically in order to mimic the body's naturally produced hormones. If you have seen Suzanne Somers in the news and/or read her books, you probably know that she is a proponent of this type of hormonal therapy. You might also remember that there was always a little confusion and controversy surrounding her theories and some debate between her and the doctors when she was on Larry King Live and 20/20. This will be discussed below, as there is scientific reasoning behind it. I like Somers' basic theory and I appreciate how far she has gone to open the eyes of American women with her healthy, holistic approach to food combining for improved digestion and for steering women away from dangerous, synthetic HRT.

"Bio -identical hormone therapy" is a term used for therapeutic hormone supplements that are molecularly identical to hormones produced by the body. Synthetic HRT, created from the molecular structures of a horse or pig, is foreign to our bodies. You still need a doctor's prescription to get bio-identical hormones and they are usually compounded (mixed by a pharmacist specifically for you) at an apothecary after the completion of your hormone testing. Depending on the type of hormone testing initially administered, your doctor's knowledge in this area, and the chosen method of delivery for the supplemented hormones, this type of hormonal therapy will often require expensive yearly testing and subsequent doctor visits to monitor it. You also may have to frequent the doctor's office due to improper dosing. Please note, this is far superior to synthetic HRT, but I do see some problems in the "model" most doctors adhere to in this type of therapy—it is often dubbed BHRT (bio-identical hormone replacement therapy).

The main issues I have seen with bio-identical hormone therapy are as follows:

Inaccurate testing may be used before prescribing.

Blood tests are often used by doctors for various types of health screenings, including hormone testing. I assume that they use blood samples for hormone testing out of convenience and familiarity. Blood tests are acceptable for certain hormone tests, but because sex hormones are fat soluble (progesterone is the most fat soluble), saliva testing is more accurate. Saliva testing will show the sex hormones (estrogen, progesterone, and testosterone) that are not bound to red blood cells (not in the serum or watery parts of the blood) and are free for the target tissues that need them. Blood testing will show mostly the sex hormones that are bound to proteins and on their way to the liver to be excreted, therefore not available to hit target cells. This inaccurate testing, coupled with a doctor who possibly lacks experience with sex hormone supplementation, can result in inconsistent dosages of hormones in the bloodstream or an overabundance of the applied hormone, which was or seemed to be originally deficient. So even though bio-identical hormones seem medically controlled as far as dosages, this is not always the case. This issue of "control of dosages" is a common complaint that the medical community often uses as a means to say that bio-identical hormone therapy cannot be easily monitored, resulting in problems over time. If you opt for this type of hormone replacement therapy, please request that your doctor uses saliva testing over the typically used blood testing, to monitor your hormone levels.

Not the best choice of hormones used or improper dosages.

Due to the occurrence of inaccurate test results, and not taking into consideration a patient's actual symptoms, women are often prescribed bio-identical estrogen and testosterone in addition to the much-needed progesterone. Supplemental estrogen and testosterone are not proven to be safe for long-term usage and are usually unnecessary, for the reasons explained earlier. In my experience, when progesterone levels are increased so that estrogen and progesterone levels become balanced, the symptoms of low energy, low libido, and low motivation (often associated with low testosterone levels) typically go away. Estrogen levels that seem low in an older postmenopausal woman can rise after a short period of time with good progesterone therapy. Therefore, at best, this extra supplemented estrogen becomes obsolete; and at worst, it can become dangerous. Many of the symptoms that might have gone away after menopause (due to drops in estrogen) that were connected to "estrogen dominance" can come back if too much estrogen is now in the body again due to supplementation that is not needed. Weight then also becomes very hard to control as estrogen will cause the body to hold on to fluid and accumulate fat. According to Dr. Lee (2006), in his book *Hormone Balance Made Simple,* "More than two thirds (66%) of women up to age 80 continue to make all the estrogen they need. Even with the ovaries removed, women make estrogen in body fat and other areas of the body. Women with plenty of body fat may make more estrogen after menopause than slim women make before menopause (pg. 20)." Most women also tend to have a weight issue at this time so extra body fat will aid temporarily until progesterone levels rise and estrogen production stays stabilized. Dr. Lee is the only one who performed long-term studies on hormone replacement in a more natural or bio-identical form (progesterone). This safer option is best explored before going on estrogen or testosterone therapy in order to diminish symptoms.

Adrenal Fatigue/Exhaustion is often not addressed when bio-identical hormone supplementation is prescribed.

An inordinate amount of stress (mental/emotional and physical), which is common for our American lifestyle, overtaxes the adrenal gland, resulting in adrenal fatigue/exhaustion (as mentioned in Chapter 1). There is a high demand for cortisol, which cannot be sustained by the body. As a result, progesterone becomes depleted as the body converts it to manufacture the cortisol it requires. This stress cycle needs to be addressed for effective hormone supplementation (especially progesterone) to take effect or the increased need for cortisol will continue to drain progesterone levels. With bio-identical hormone therapy, the conversion of progesterone to cortisol is not properly addressed. The progesterone given in this therapy will convert to cortisol while the estrogen and testosterone supplementation given increases the levels of those hormones, perhaps leaving you in worse shape due to exacerbating your original imbalance. I have seen this many times in my center. If your symptoms are not gone, your doctor has not hit the nail on the head no matter what your lab results say!

Holistic practitioners who administer bio-identical therapy may prescribe herbal supplements in order to aid the adrenal gland. Oral (pill) forms of DHEA can help to alleviate some of the stress on the adrenal gland and allow it to rebuild. DHEA enables the adrenal gland to better handle the increased demand for cortisol and is actually a good concept. However, because most "stressed out" Americans suffer from poor digestion; these oral forms of therapy rarely solve adrenal fatigue/exhaustion. Most ingredients will not be properly assimilated, and the issue of drained progesterone remains, leaving estrogen and testosterone levels too high in comparison to progesterone. I will further explain a simple and effective adrenal support method in Chapter 8.

Poor delivery system used for hormone supplementation.

Bio-identical therapy is most often times delivered through a cream, which is to be rubbed into the skin. If the delivery system your doctor/pharmacist chooses for this therapy is not a true "trans-dermal" (going directly into the bloodstream through the skin) delivery system, the hormones can build up in the body's fatty tissue over the course of several months and then drop into the system inconsistently, like a sponge that has been oversaturated. When hormones are administered through a cream and rubbed into the "fatty" areas of the body, using a "rotating body-part" method of application, the delivery system is often alcohol- based. This allows the hormones to go directly into the fatty tissues and saturate them before ever getting into the blood stream. This commonly happens when supplementing with progesterone; so, be aware of any progesterone cream from the Internet or health food store that requires you to "rotate" application sites. Often, this will result in inconsistent dosages of the hormone in the bloodstream or, eventually over months of use, an overabundance of the applied hormone, which was originally deficient. Even though these hormones seem medically controlled as far as dosage is concerned, this is often not the case. During the first several months of the treatment with this type of bio-identical hormone therapy cream, the symptoms will often go away, but if there is a buildup of hormones (even progesterone), over time, all of your symptoms will come back. This is where the controversy lies over this type of hormone therapy. People do not seem to understand this concept so they are confused as to whether or not the hormone therapy worked at all. One of the doctors who challenged Suzanne Somers asked a question of this nature . . . *If bio-identical hormones are so great, then why do medical doctors see so many of these women back in their offices nine to twelve months later with the return of all their original symptoms?* This doctor had a point, and the reason is due to "build up." As I mentioned earlier, too much of something in the body can demonstrate the same symptoms as not enough. This applies to progesterone, the good and safe hormone, as well. If your levels are low and you supplement with bio-identical therapy, you will get relief. However, if the delivery system is incorrect, your symptoms will gradually return as progesterone builds up in the fatty tissue, which may turn you off from trying to get relief through any type of hormone supplementation. A sublingual form of progesterone is much better if using bio-identical therapy or a true "trans-dermal" cream (see Chapter 8).

In addition to the above, keep the following in mind;

According to the American College of Obstetricians and Gynecologists (2005): Most compounded products, including bio-identical hormones, have not undergone rigorous clinical testing for either safety or efficacy. Also, there are concerns regarding the purity, potency, and quality of compounded products. In 2001, the FDA analyzed a variety of 29 product samples from 12 compounding pharmacies and found that 34% of them failed one or more standard quality tests. Additionally, 9 of the 10 failing products failed assay or potency tests, with all containing less of the active ingredient than expected.

The above statement, though accurate, kind of makes me chuckle because most medically affiliated organizations are usually proponents of synthetic drugs even though there are approximately 106,000 deaths per year from misuse of synthetic drugs. This statistic is from the groundbreaking 2003 medical report, *Death by Medicine,* by Drs. Gary Null, Carolyn Dean, Martin Feldman, Debora Rasio, and Dorothy Smith. Oftentimes, the side effects of the birth control pill and synthetic hormones are "played down" by certain organizations and pharmaceutical companies in order to promote their use. Otherwise, no one in their right mind would ever take them. When watching their commercials, have you ever really heard what they are saying while the beautiful young woman is prancing around the screen living a care-free life? The possible side effects are pretty bad! Now these organizations are banding together to overemphasize the risks of the somewhat healthier alternative of bio-identical hormones. In my opinion, the logic behind this argument needs to make more sense for me to be able to swallow it. They must first admit how dangerous their options are in order to be able to say that these bio-identical options are "just as risky." I feel that they should be more concerned with women's health and more eager to explain just how dangerous synthetic hormones can be. This would then make them more credible when they speak on any issues with bio- identical hormone methods.

Even though study after study has proven synthetic hormones to be unsafe, from all my experience, the model of bio-identical hormone therapy, although much safer, still has some issues to be worked out. If you do decide to supplement with bio-identical hormones, please be sure to get saliva testing done beforehand and then biannually to monitor hormone levels, to prevent buildup in the fatty tissues.

Due to the above stated reasons, I do not recommend the bio-identical model of hormone replacement therapy to my clients but prefer natural hormone balancing.

Risks of Too Much Estrogen (Synthetic or Bio-Identical) as We Age

Once in menopause, or following a full hysterectomy (removal of a woman's ovaries and uterus), there is no more "ovarian" estrogen available, so our body turns to our adrenal source of estrogen. Even if you lead a very stressful life and are now in "second-level depletion" of the adrenal gland (DHEA is low so this source of estrogen is depleted as well), you can still have optimal estrogen production, for the reasons explained below. "There has yet to be a study proving the relationship between estrogen deficiency and menopausal symptoms or related diseases." This was pointed out by Dr. Jerilynn Prior, professor of endocrinology at the University in Vancouver B.C. Canada (Lee, 2004, p. 44).

As explained in Dr. Lee's (2004) book, *What Your Doctor May Not Tell You About Menopause*, the body also has the ability to use estrone—a weaker, less active, and safer form of estrogen, which is often produced from the fat cells and the skin cells after menopause (p. 38). Estrone can take over the decreased production of estradiol, which was the main estrogen made in the ovaries prior to menopause. Estradiol is twelve times more potent than estrone, and in the presence of adequate progesterone, estradiol will often be converted to estrone sulfate, an essentially inactive form that is stored mainly in the fat cells for later use as needed. Progesterone also induces the production of an enzyme used to convert estradiol to estrone. This seems to be a natural checks-and-balances system to be sure natural estrogen does not get too high, which could eventually cause diseases like breast cancer. This is not the case when a woman takes the birth control pill (see Chapter or synthetic estrogen (for example, Premarin), as these high levels of synthetic estrogen take a toll on the body as it tries to stay in balance—despite drained progesterone levels.

I believe that the rise in breast cancer in more modern societies, like our own, is the result of the toll that stress has played on lowering our protective progesterone levels, the use of synthetic hormones, the impact of xenoestrogens (see Chapter 5), and our poor diet. These factors are all unique to our country and this is why we have a higher incidence of female- related cancers than other less developed countries. Progesterone is a key necessity in avoiding hormone-sensitive breast cancers since it suppresses (down regulates) estrogen receptors in breast tissue. (I am only addressing this type of breast cancer here, as there are other complicated factors in other forms of this disease.)

My former colleague and I performed our own preliminary breast cancer study (Appendix B) using saliva testing to examine hormone patterns in women with estrogen receptor positive (ER+) breast cancer. The study has since been published since the first edition of this book (*Original Internist*, Sept 2012). The study looked at the most obvious pattern first: the specific ratio of estrogen to progesterone. From there, we looked at the ratios of the three main estrogens to determine which one might be elevated with hormone sensitive cancers so that we could establish a possible relationship. In my direct experience, women with breast cancer always have imbalanced sex hormones.

The goal of the study was to show trends in saliva hormonal profiles of women with ER+ positive breast cancer. These trends could then serve as an early indicator of potential breast cancer when compared with a new patient's saliva test results. The simple version of the results indicated that all of the women showed a poor estrogen to progesterone ratio, meaning they were all "estrogen dominant."

One study cited in the *American Journal of Epidemiology*, by Dr. Linda D. Cowan, found that women with progesterone deficiency had 5.4 times the risk of pre-menopausal breast cancer, while a Mayo Clinic study showed that women with a history of progesterone deficiency as evidenced by symptoms such as irregular periods had 3.6 times the risk of postmenopausal cancer. This further establishes that there are trends to be observed with women who get breast cancer.

Dr. Reiss (2001), author of *Natural Hormone Balance for Women* agrees with this same concept of the "progesterone protection factor" by showing the conversion of estradiol (E2) into estrone (E1), which is a form of estrogen that is 85% weaker than estradiol. This conversion can only take place in the presence of progesterone, coupled with a specific enzyme. This again shows that progesterone is involved in converting excess estrogen into a safer form.

The important point to take from this section is that any woman who has breast cancer has imbalanced sex hormones. No medical doctor in the United States can disprove this fact. I only wish, with all the billions of dollars raised by breast cancer awareness organizations, that this point would be part of the education process. Education is power and with this dreaded disease it offers hope.

Basic Health Tips to Balance Female Hormones and Decrease Chances of Female-Related Cancers:

- Keep progesterone levels up by augmenting with a natural progesterone cream (such as the one described in Chapter 8). Dosing can be based on saliva testing or a symptom-based protocol under a professional's guidance.

- Consider an adrenal supplement to reduce the conversion of progesterone to cortisol. (See Chapter 8 for information on the supplement that I use in my heath center).

- Assess physical stress in your life (all types) and lower these factors by increasing the number of hours you sleep, lowering pain with spinal adjustments and by reducing your intake of processed food and foods you are sensitive to. Common sensitive foods are dairy- based and wheat-based products which tend to cause gas, bloating, stomach pain, or weight gain.

- Assess mental/emotional stress caused by your daily schedule, relationships, your job, self-esteem, or suppressed emotions. (Read about practical ways to do this in Chapter 8).

- Take twenty to thirty minutes daily to relieve stress. This will "open your valve" so it does not all blow up on some innocent person like your husband or a co-worker. Use a meditation CD, if necessary, to relax your brainwave patterns to a less stressed state. (Read more in Chapter 8).

- Eat cruciferous vegetables (like broccoli and cabbage) everyday. Cruciferous vegetables are chock full of nutrients that can help to protect you from developing breast cancer as they affect the conversion of more potent estrogen (estradiol) to weaker, less active estrogen (estrone) so it is not as active and therefore less harmful.

To get a full 16 page report of studies showing how natural hormone balancing can reduce the risk of estrogen receptor positive breast center, please email info@bebalancedcenters.com. The report is called, *"The BeBalanced Approach to Breast Cancer."*

Balance Can Be Smooth and Simple

Menopause is a natural shift that all women must eventually go through. A woman can look and feel her best in her menopausal years. This is the time that her children have grown, she may have the opportunity to retire, and she can actually enjoy a more relaxed life

After a hysterectomy or menopause there can be a smooth transition from a woman's main source of estrogen from the ovaries (mainly estradiol) to the estrogen that comes from the fat (estrone), with no real gaps in the production. Therefore, the idea of supplementing with more estrogen does not have to be entertained and the need for dangerous synthetic hormones can be eradicated. However, this smooth transition into menopause can only happen if a woman has normal levels of progesterone. If progesterone levels are in the normal range; then and only then, can menopause be a symptom-free life transition. In most cases though, as I have explained, progesterone levels are usually deficient due to excess stressors and other factors. Therefore, if you pass through to menopause and your progesterone levels have been low for a long time, then your estrogen levels from the fat and skin never get the opportunity to "kick in." The end result can be lowered estrogen levels, progesterone levels bottoming out, and an era of new uncomfortable postmenopausal symptoms such as vaginal dryness (that leads to painful intercourse), low libido, low energy, dry skin, hair loss, and brittle nails.

When natural hormone balancing occurs through addressing adrenal fatigue/exhaustion and by supplementing progesterone, ovulation can return to normal and a monthly period often returns for younger women who experienced pre-mature menopausal symptoms. However, the periods are light, normal, and symptom-free. Some women are annoyed by this return of menstruation, but the benefits of becoming symptom free when estrogen and progesterone are balanced outweigh a brief period each month.

The body seems to simply concern itself with birth, development, childbearing capacity, and then death. We do not look at life this way, of course. Once the childbearing years are over, we look forward to the freedom to have fun, vacation, and retire. Unfortunately, the "golden" years are often wrought with so many annoying symptoms that we feel like throwing in the towel! When hormone levels get low, the body senses the inability to procreate and stops putting so much effort into its survival. When hormone levels are balanced and return to optimal levels with the right kind of supplementation, the body acts as if it were younger and revs back up, even at this stage of life.

To recap, the common menopausal treatments used today are neither safe nor very effective. The synthetic approach to fix these symptoms such as HRT is more of a bandage approach, which only masks symptoms at best and can be dangerous at worst. Plus, there are no other benefits of being fully balanced. The bio-identical approach is more of a silver bullet that aims to increase any specific lowered hormone seen on a saliva test (like estrogen and testosterone) but does not address the real cause; adrenal fatigue and lowered progesterone levels. When these two areas are fixed, the other more "risky" hormones are not required as a treatment method. At best, the bio-identical approach provides temporary relief, and at worse it can contribute to the overall imbalance; therefore, all symptoms never go away. Also, there is always some danger as having too much estrogen, which can spark female-related cancers, as well as stubborn weight gain around the midsection. This approach can be much more effective if simple modifications are made such as those mentioned in this chapter; use saliva testing, address adrenal issues, and implement a proper delivery system to avoid buildup. These suggestions, along with progesterone therapy, should all be implemented before moving forward with riskier estrogen and testosterone supplementation.

I feel that the most conservative, but effective approach, is to work with the body using natural and safe progesterone supplementation, and addressing adrenal issues with small diet and lifestyle changes. This will allow hormones to stay balanced throughout the course of our lives and we can experience a higher long-term quality of life. Another benefit of natural hormone balancing is the anti-aging factor. Once sex hormones are truly balanced and overall stress hormones are low, bone loss is dramatically reduced or even eliminated, cholesterol will not rise, blood pressure will be reduced, anxiety and depression will diminish, and sleep is deepened.

I like to say, "With proper hormone balance, weight goes, age slows, and vitality grows." Life is a journey. Through natural hormonal balance, you can improve the quality of this journey. Hopefully, you now understand that you do not have to choose between feeling great and being safe!

CHAPTER 3

The Hormone Shift & Weight

The Use of Glandular Therapy and Ketosis to Lose Stubborn Weight...

Why is it so hard to lose weight after the age of forty?

Is the "calories in-calories out" philosophy valid when it fails in many cases?

Why can some women manage their weight easily while others cannot?

How can cardiovascular exercise actually cause weight gain when certain imbalances are present?

Solution: Temporarily engage in a low calorie, ketogenic/ glandular protocol to rebalance the brain's orchestration of hormones for efficient weight loss at any age.

Specifics on a natural hormone balancing solution (refer to Chapter 8)

Have you ever wondered if obesity is genetic, or if age-related weight gain is inevitable—as popular opinion suggests? The answer to both of these questions is a resounding, "No!" Anyone who has problems managing their weight always has some type of underlying hormonal imbalance. When you balance the hormones first as a foundation, fast and effective weight loss can be achieved at any age.

In my experience, the hormone levels of an obese or overweight person have always shift ed in some way to a state of imbalance. Lifestyle and dietary factors aside; insulin imbalances, thyroid problems, and out-of- whack sex and stress hormone levels, in some combination, are always a factor in an obese person. The question is, "Which comes first?" Does the hormonal imbalance affect our behavior (impede energy and motivation for workouts and create intense cravings for processed/

sugar-laden foods), causing weight gain? Or, is it our behavior (inactive lifestyle coupled with the consumption of sugar/processed foods) that causes the hormonal imbalance, promoting weight gain?

We may not solve that mystery here, but truthfully, it is probably a little bit of both. When trying to aid an obese person, the medical community and the fitness industry fail to address imbalanced sex and stress hormones, which are the heart of the problem. For some overweight people, even strict adherence to a healthy diet and exercise program can prove disappointing. Hence, there is a growing population of women who seem to gain weight around menopause or find it virtually impossible to lose weight at this stage of their life. This group of women often feels that no one—doctors and personal trainers included—can help them or even understand the challenges they are facing. Sure, with age, weight may get a little harder to control, but that is usually because the underlying issues are not addressed and they tend to worsen with time, as any sort of degenerative condition does. Remember, it is not simply time, but rather abuse (or an imbalance) over the course of time that will cause stubborn excess weight gain.

Simply put, the hormonal imbalance between estrogen and progesterone, due to stress and the increased demand for cortisol (as described in Chapter 1), needs to be addressed for successful weight loss in pre-menopausal, peri-menopausal and menopausal women. Also important to note, "estrogen dominance" is often associated with high insulin levels in the bloodstream. This condition will cause blood sugar and insulin imbalances over time, exacerbating the problem. While the stubborn fat seems to be related to age, I have seen many young women and even adolescents, with hormonal imbalances, struggle with weight issues. An example of this is the growing group of adolescent girls with PCOS (polycystic ovarian syndrome) characterized by insulin imbalances and the inability to ovulate. Therefore, we cannot say that hormonal imbalances are always related to our age. This dispels the notion that age alone is connected to stubborn fat being deposited. The issue of weight is tied to the hormonal imbalance. I will make this point; however, weight issues tend to get worse as you age, especially if you have had a hormonal imbalance your whole life.

This leads us to a few more questions. Are there genetic markers for obesity? Sure! If you have one, do you have to be obese? No! Genetic predispositions often need to be triggered by a variety of lifestyle factors. There are people who do not get cancer, even though they have a genetic encoding for it. This is because there have to be other lifestyle factors involved as well. Certainly, a person genetically predisposed to a condition would have more of a likelihood of forming that condition. However, the way I look at it is; they are not usually predisposed to the actual condition, like "obesity," but more to the underlying hormonal imbalance connected to it (examples: low progesterone). So, if we cannot totally blame genetics for weight gain/obesity, then other factors in a person's lifestyle most likely need to be addressed. In doing this, however, we need to go a little bit deeper than the "calories-in, calories-out" philosophy on obesity and look at subclinical conditions that lead to weight gain. This "further digging" into other causes of weight gain became necessary to me when I saw many women who were following a clean, healthy diet and active lifestyle, but were not able to budge their weight . . . *I was one of them!*

The message that I am presenting here should offer relief and hope because it puts more power and some responsibility in your hands. I believe that we are not victims here on this earth but co-creators of many of the circumstances and situations in our lives, including diseased "states." I believe everything has a cause and effect whether we can clearly see it or not, and this is all governed by specific laws of nature that cannot be broken, nor can exceptions be made.

From reading Chapters 1 and 2, you can see how important hormone balance is to looking and feeling your best. PMS and menopausal symptoms fade when adrenal fatigue/exhaustion is addressed and natural progesterone in the body is raised. Natural progesterone also buffers blood sugar to aid in weight loss by tempering estrogen's influence on insulin. Theoretically, rebalancing the hormones will help a woman with a stubborn weight issue shed body fat and excess fluid. Those who previously struggled will finally be able to lose one to two pounds per week while adhering to a healthy, lower-calorie diet, and an adequate exercise program (resistance training is best). Just on a "relief of symptoms" basis alone, it makes sense that a woman would be able to lose weight due to the fact that she will likely stick with a healthy diet and exercise program when her mood is lifted (decrease in anxiety/depression symptoms), her energy is increased, and her motivation and willpower is increased. These are all common good side effects of having balanced female hormones (estrogen and progesterone) and lowered stress hormones (cortisol).

However, it became very apparent to me after years of experience that even after women would balance their estrogen and progesterone, and be virtually free of sleep, mood, and other female "issues," that oftentimes many women still struggle with losing stubborn fat once they hit the age of thirty five or forty. This was definitely the case with me, so I was determined to find an answer. Results from regular diet and exercise, which should now be more effective with the sex hormones balanced, still came much too slowly for this group of peri-menopausal or menopausal women, making it hard for them to stay compliant long enough to reach their goal weight. I learned that for this group of women, with pre-existing hormone imbalances, even cardiovascular exercise, especially done in a linear fashion (such as running, EFX machine, Stairmasters, etc.), will actually increase cortisol levels in the body. The brain views this "exercise" as a stress, like you are running away from a wild animal, and will increase cortisol, which will then further lower progesterone (as you learned in Chapter 1). This makes weight loss impossible! Please do not think I am discouraging "movement," as we all sit too much in America. I really recommend dance instead because it moves your body outside the normal linear planes of walking and running and serves as a great way to "unwind." Dance, which can be much more fun than running, is much better for the joints and muscles and does not evoke the stress response. I advocate dance if any cardiovascular work is desired, but feel your heart gets a workout with yoga or other resistance training of any kind. Resistance training though is really essential as we age and keeps your metabolism up and keeps you looking firm and strong. This can be done with weights, bands, kettle balls, body weight, power yoga or even core work like Pilates. At my center, we stress this type of ongoing exercise after we get women's hormones balanced and their stubborn fat off as you will see coming up.

You can hopefully see why women who are trying to depend on doing cardiovascular exercise alone to lose weight at this age, are left extremely frustrated. It is essential that hormones be balanced for stubborn weight to be lose initially and then resistance training can help keep us strong as we age and aid in maintaining our new weight.

My goal in delving deeper into the hormonal connection to weight loss was to help women lose weight quickly and feel great (hormonally) while they are losing weight, so that motivation to be compliant to the program is not an issue. This increases dedication to implementing healthy lifestyle advice afterward, to maintain their new figure and have a renewed lease on life!

This took a bit more than just looking at what I will call the "lower" glands of the body such as the adrenal glands, pancreas, ovaries, or thyroid. From my experience, when these glands have been overtaxed for a longer time, due to chronic stress, the hormonal orchestration system would be scrambled and not running smoothly. After all, in a finely tuned orchestra, if three of the seven instruments are not keeping the same tempo as the rest of the instruments, it throws off the whole symphony. At some point you have to look at the conductor and say, "What is going on here?" He has been watching and listening the entire time, knowing where things went awry. We will call this conductor the hypothalamus, a gland in the brain that oversees hormone function as mentioned in Chapter 1.

Let us now go a bit deeper into how the hypothalamus operates. It is the vital part of the brain that controls the autonomic nervous system, which is responsible for maintaining the homeostasis, or balance, of the body. Damage to the hypothalamus will result in many severe imbalances to the internal environment of the body. The hypothalamus is directly linked to the thirst center, hunger center, the body's thermostat, and circadian rhythms. Damage to the hypothalamus will frequently cause water, glucose, and temperature imbalances, as well as throwing off the timing of the release of certain hormones. The workings of this process are described as "feedback loops." The hypothalamus releases certain hormones that stimulate the pituitary gland (known as the master endocrine gland) to release other hormones into the body that will actually stimulate glands such as the thyroid gland, adrenal gland, pancreas, ovaries, etc. When levels of those hormones are adequate in the bloodstream, a feedback loop system senses this and the hypothalamus stops stimulating the pituitary to release hormones to stimulate those glands. Then, when hormone levels get low, the hypothalamus is warned to then increase production of its hormones that affect the pituitary.

Since the hypothalamus controls the pituitary gland, it obviously oversees the orchestration of the entire hormonal production in the body. It is vitally important to understand that the nervous system is directly controlled by the hypothalamus. The nervous system has authority to stimulate glands to release sugar and adrenaline for "fight or flight" response. This is essential because outside stimulation, or even danger (perceived or real), by our conscious mind needs to be factored into the brain's ability to direct our hormones. The hypothalamus serves as an important bridge between the emotions (what we sense, see, hear, and feel from the environment) and our physiological responses, such as going into the "fight or flight" mode. When we are upset because we are stuck in traffic but there is no life or death issue, the body still perceives this as stress and the heart rate increases, the blood flows to the skeletal muscles, etc. Our prehistoric minds cannot discern the difference between life altering stress and day-to-day irritating situations. There needs to be a link between our emotions (our minds' perception) and how our body prepares for the action needed to sustain itself. This bridge is the hypothalamus, which is now being studied for its connection to weight, via the stress and weight gain connection.

The delicate balance of these hormonal systems, directed by the hypothalamus, directly affects body weight and fat storage, even to the point where some scientists believe that the specific set point for your weight can be thrown off by damage to the hypothalamus. Washington University School of Medicine confers how the hypothalamus maintains the body's functions at a regular level called the "set point," which acts as a biochemical thermostat, maintaining bodily functions within a narrow set of parameters. In a recent article on hypothalamic dysfunction by the Maryland Medical Center, it states that the hypothalamus influences the pituitary, which in turn influences the thyroid, which is a major controller of our metabolism.

There is obviously no quick, simple test that can be done at your doctor's office to see if the hypothalamus is working optimally, nor would your typical family doctor, nutritionist, personal trainer even think to look here in dealing with your frustration over the inability to lose weight. Therefore, it leaves many women frustrated because their endocrinologist will simply focus on simple blood sugar imbalances, and offer drugs such as *Metformin* or insulin, or test the thyroid levels which are often initially still within range of "normal," therefore no synthetic thyroid medication can be offered, and you are sent away bewildered and discouraged. OBGYN doctors do understand hormones, but more from a perspective of female disease, pregnancy, childbirth, and breast-feeding. Likely, the birth control pill, or in-office procedures are offered as the solution for any type of female symptoms, and weight is often not even addressed. Unfortunately, the least informed on the stubborn weight loss issue connected to hormones is often your general medical practitioner or family doctor. Oftentimes they will just instruct you to just eat less and exercise more, or even possibly take an antidepressant if you are "that upset" about your weight. If you are not feeling supported and heard by the medical community, the problem can become extremely frustrating.

In researching more on this fascinating part of the brain called the hypothalamus, I was introduced to the work of the brilliant Dr. A.T.W. Simeons, and his research on how the hypothalamus plays a strong role in metabolism. Simeons spearheaded this concept of the hypothalamus being an integral part of blood sugar balance, metabolism, and weight. He found that obese people have damage to the hypothalamus, often causing it to not function properly. The main things he observed were that obese people seemed to share certain traits: intense physical hunger, a slow metabolism, an intense desire to eat when not hungry, abnormally high food cravings, and the issue of constantly storing fat in "abnormal" areas of the body (hips, stomach, and thighs). His work led him to believe that an individual could be born with a genetic weakness of the hypothalamus, and a traumatic event could overtax and damage the hypothalamus any time in life, or an individual can slowly damage the hypothalamus over time with intense emotional stress or an over consumption of sugar-laden refined foods. He learned that in some cases this damage to the hypothalamus could be mild, and the individual would slowly, over time, store fat in the hip, stomach, and thighs. The damage varies in severity, and can be determined by how quickly a person gains weight and how difficult it is for them to shed the weight.

Dr. Simeons was ridiculed by many doctors back in his day as well as doctors in America today. I find this fascinating because no one seems to have the "cure" for obesity in their pocket, nor has any drug company cornered the market on this epidemic problem. I think he was the closest to being on to something. His theory is even reflected in current research studies, such as one by Dr. Michael W Schwartz, who is the director of The Diabetes and Obesity Center of Excellence at the University of Washington in Seattle. Schwartz notes that the brain; originally connected to glucose metabolism, was simply not the primary focus when the discovery of insulin came about in the 1920s. His paper states that all treatment for diabetes intended to increase insulin levels, or increase insulin sensitivity. Schwartz suggests there is an underlying cause of diabetes that deals with the brain, and that in both animal and human studies there is a strong indication that there is a brain center regulatory system on blood glucose levels that is totally independent of the actions of the hormone insulin. Surprisingly, fifty percent of normal glucose uptake is connected to this brain mechanism, and research says that the impairment of the brain center system is common, and causes more burden to be placed on the pancreatic system to compensate for this. When this occurs, the pancreas needs to overproduce insulin, and this can throw off the brain-centered mechanism. So begins a vicious cycle, eventually ending in diabetes. Dr. Swartz suggests that an approach which targets insulin levels, as well as the brain, would be optimal and the latest research is going in this direction. This makes sense, based on the fact that a stressful thought, not just ingesting sugar, will cause a hormonal cascade that results in insulin being released.

As you initially learned in Chapter 1, when we are under constant stress, cortisol rises. In addition, along with this rise in cortisol, the body also releases stored blood sugar from the muscles, called glycogen, so we have energy for "fight or flight." Always following this release of blood sugar is a corresponding release of insulin, to get the blood sugar into the cells. When we are under constant stress, we have constant sugar and constant insulin releasing into the bloodstream. Over time, this can cause an over- demand for insulin causing the body to need more of it to be effective - a common condition called "insulin resistance" as well as increases fat storage (Figure 3-1).

Figure 3-1
The Effect of Stress on Blood Sugar and Fat Storage

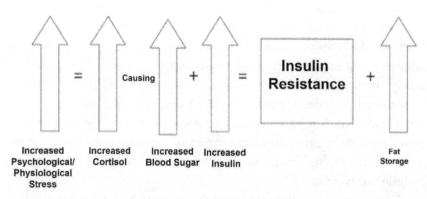

This is the very same reaction in the body as consuming too much sugar. Elevated blood sugar levels and "insulin resistance" are connected to weight gain, cravings, and increased appetite, which the hypothalamus has control over. Simply stated, when you are under stress and cortisol rises, the body always follows by releasing stored sugar into the bloodstream, then insulin follows to bring down blood sugar and to get the sugar into the cells. So how can we say that diabetes or pre-diabetes (commonly known as "insulin resistance") is only a mechanism of a failed pancreas, without looking at the cause of the constant demand for insulin, which is causing the pancreas's demise? This is a very myopic way of looking at the problem. Unfortunately, this is very common for most of American medical doctors.

This all shows that Dr. Simeons was really onto something back then, with his "hypothalamus" theory of seemingly unexplained weight gain. This theory; however, was based on years of observations while working with obese patients in Europe. He was convinced that the hypothalamus was the key to optimal weight. Later, while spending time in Africa, he noted that malnourished pregnant women still gave birth to healthy babies! This is due to the body's ability to utilize the stomach, hip, and thigh fat to nourish the baby, due to a hormone called hCG (human chorionic gonadotropin). This led to him becoming the doctor most famously connected with the use of hCG, known as the "pregnancy hormone," for weight loss. The name seems to fit, because hCG rises dramatically in a pregnant woman. This hormone allows the woman's body fat to be used as a source of stored energy if she were to ever be low on calories (starving), and needed it to feed her unborn baby.

Part of Dr. Simeon's theory was that a major catastrophic stressful event would seem to throw off the hypothalamus in its regulation of hunger or fat storing. He also noted that the hypothalamus can be slowly thrown off over time with chronic stress and poor eating. If your thoughts alone, or perception of a situation, can affect your blood sugar and insulin release/demand in preparation for "fight or flight," your stressful thoughts over time can cause "insulin resistance," which affects your weight. The mind truly affects the body, and this does not exclude our weight.

Another way to look at this vicious cycle is to understand that when sugar is constantly high in the bloodstream, either due to cortisol being elevated from your mental /emotional stress, or from you consuming sugar, caffeine or alcohol, you have the tendency to become "insulin resistant," and therefore only burn sugar, without the ability to burn fat efficiently. A simple way to understand "insulin resistance" is to think of it in terms of the following example. If you had a neighbor that would come to your front door and bring you some treats, you would be happy to see him and let him in the door. But if your neighbor was constantly coming over and always hanging around outside your door, you would then start to become resistant to letting him in, just due to being tired of seeing him so often. This can be a good comparison for when insulin is constantly "hanging out" in the bloodstream outside of your cells. Initially, insulin helps allow sugar to get into your cells, but after a while your cells become resistant to allowing the insulin to do its job. When you become "insulin resistant," your body needs more and more insulin to do the same job of getting sugar into your cells. In this case, your neighbor would need to bring you bigger and better gifts if you're going to keep letting him inside your door. The condition of "insulin resistance" should be taken seriously, because it paves the way for diabetes, and often occurs for decades before this disease develops. With "insulin resistance," the pancreas is in a hyper state of overproducing insulin, due to demands. How long this can go on will vary depending upon each person's genetics; I believe, since one can be born with a genetically weak organ. When the pancreas can no longer sustain this output of insulin, the pancreas is in a hypo state in which less insulin is produced, leaving blood sugar high -specifically after meals, but also affecting fasting blood sugar levels. As I mentioned in Chapter 1, the adrenal gland is hyper, and then hypo, as I will mention in Chapter 4, on the thyroid gland going hyper and then hypo, you will note a trend with the body's glands. Stress causes most glands to be hyper until they can no longer maintain homeostasis that way, and then their production of the hormone goes low. Obviously, either extreme is not good.

When the pancreas is in a fully hypo state for a long time, you usually develop diabetes. This needs to be treated with either medication or insulin, if hormones are not balanced or your diet is not drastically changed. The high insulin levels that have been occurring over time leading up to diabetes are associated with abdominal weight gain, cholesterol abnormalities, and high blood pressure, commonly wrapped into one condition called Metabolic Syndrome or "Syndrome X." Sadly, almost all adults in our modern-day society have some degree of "insulin resistance," and in women it is even more common.

Things get much more complicated with blood sugar for women, and even more complicated closer to menopause when progesterone levels really fall and estrogen is very dominant. Progesterone helps balance blood sugar, so when this hormone is low there are more rises and falls in blood sugar, and the tendency for hypoglycemia and the resulting cravings. I'm sure I do not need to remind you of the vicious cycle that would occur with blood sugar if we indulge these cravings and have the pretzels, chocolate, or soda.

Estrogen is now being studied more in-depth for its connection with blood sugar. Most American women experience an "estrogen dominance" condition, which often will cause an over stimulation of the pancreas by acting directly on the beta cells to make them resistant to death, and to increase insulin production. This can be beneficial in helping the pancreatic cells to adapt to higher insulin demands, such as pregnancy or breast-feeding. However, extreme or long-term "estrogen dominance," or estrogen stimulation with estrogen mimicking chemicals, can actually cause "insulin resistance" by exhausting beta cells through overstimulation. This is what is going on with most American women, and why a high percentage of them who are in a severe case of "estrogen dominance" and progesterone deficiency (with elevated cortisol levels) cannot easily get into or stay in a ketogenic (fat burning) state, commonly induced by diets like the Atkins diet. Please bear with me while I get a little technical here. Estrogen increases the liver's insulin sensitivity by decreasing something called gluconeogenesis (energy production from non- carbohydrate carbon substrates such as pyruvate, lactate, etc.) Lactate and pyruvate are the byproducts of the body using fat for energy from a normal ketogenic diet. So if you ever tried the Atkins diet or any ketogenic diet, which often promotes fast fat loss in men, and you urinated on a keto stick to see if you had these byproducts to show "ketosis," and the stick did not turn color, this is the reason. In short, estrogen prevents the body from going easily into a fat burning or ketogenic state, using fat as the primary source of fuel. This is the problem that many women face, and the more out of balance or "estrogen dominant" they get, the worst the problem is, and they lose hope.

One reason I strongly suggest progesterone supplementation is to balance out estrogen, which allows for a more natural fat burning state in a woman's body. Lacking progesterone, which has that balancing effect on blood sugar, makes the problem of "insulin resistance" synergistically worse. One medical study, conducted in England in 1993, found that as high as 67% of diabetic women reported premenstrual syndrome changes in their blood sugar levels and up to 70% reported changes in their blood sugar during menstruation. These changes seemed more prevalent in women who also suffer from other premenstrual symptoms. This is just one study that would validate the roller coaster effect that estrogen has on blood sugar via insulin. As a matter of fact, blood sugar fluctuations due to physical (sugar, caffeine, alcohol) or psychological stresses are a more modern day problem, and cause an increased stress load on the body as it tries to maintain homeostasis. This results in mood swings, irritability, anxiety, insomnia, cravings, and of course weight gain. High cortisol and a simple sex hormone imbalance are always tied to this scenario in the body.

Men can become "insulin resistant" over time as well, but tend not to have the same proclivity for this issue as women that are hormonally out of balance. The first imbalance that needs to be corrected for women to lose fat efficiently is the estrogen/progesterone balance. This will result in progesterone rising as stress is reduced, and the need for the stress hormone, cortisol, goes down. The next step for actual fat/weight loss though for women over forty is to be sure that blood sugar is balanced, and that the body becomes more sensitive to insulin, so that a woman can burn her stored body fat. From my experience, in our day and age with all the stress that we are under, the only way to do this is by generating a ketogenic state. Ketosis is simply a state where the body burns fat instead of sugar for energy. Ketones are a needed and essential healing energy source in our cells that come from the normal metabolism of fat.

Dr. Gabriela Segura states in *The Health Matrix* that the entire body uses ketones in a more safe and effective way than the energy coming from carbohydrates or sugar (glucose). She notes that our bodies will, in fact, produce enough ketones (fuel) when we eat less than 60 g of carbs per day and by eating a very low-carb diet or no carbs at all (like a caveman), we can actually become keto-adapted.

Burning fat is a much more efficient source of fuel, with fat having nine calories per gram as opposed to carbohydrates which have five calories per gram. Carbohydrates were meant to be burned for short burst of energy back in prehistoric times, since the breaking down of fat takes a little longer and a few more steps in the cell. Carbohydrates were meant to be the initial energy used when fighting, running away, or sprinting to catch an animal, etc. Fat was fuel for day-to-day, long-term sustaining activities like running the body or doing daily work. I believe a hypothalamic disorder, as I addressed above, throws this off in our modern society. We no longer can get to our adequate reserves of stored body fat to burn it off between meals and while we sleep at night. This is due to us having elevated levels of cortisol and blood sugar in our modern society, causing "insulin resistance."

Hopefully now you understand the unique relationship between insulin and cortisol. Cortisol is actually directing your cells to become resistant to the normal action of insulin or causing "insulin resistance." Dr. Cynthia Shelby-Lane, a board-certified, anti-aging of functional medicine specialist, explains that cortisol is actually a balancing hormone for insulin. This means that if insulin is out of balance, cortisol will also be out of balance. She states that if you have a large demand for cortisol, due to your body's attempt to balance insulin, you also will not be able to balance your estrogen and progesterone ratios.

So in review, too much stress or too much sugar over time will lead to "insulin resistance," and this will cause you to store fat. Ideally, insulin is to get sugar into your muscles for you to burn as energy, but when sugar is in excess, the fat cells begin to fill with fat. Besides, our muscles can only hold so much stored sugar (glycogen). When capacity is full the body has no choice but to store excess sugar as fat.

During this process of extra sugar in the bloodstream, we simply burn the sugar that is in our blood stream which has been released from the fight or flight response. This, in my opinion, is not how it was meant to be. Going into a healthy ketogenic state, I believe, is going back to where the body wants to be. The heart and the kidneys actually prefer ketone bodies to burn as fuel as opposed to carbohydrates. When the body is in a state of ketosis and burning off stored body fat, the person's blood sugar remains constant. This is very soothing to the mood and to the internal stress of the body.

We always need to factor into all of this the extremely high demand for cortisol in women due to our modern society and all the multi-tasking we do. It is easy to understand from Chapter 1 that if you meditate, do yoga, or get a massage, you will lower stress in your body, and therefore lower the demands for stress hormone like cortisol. It is equally important to change your diet to stabilize your blood sugar and insulin in order to lower cortisol demands as well. Actually, this may be even more important, and thankfully one thing we have control over, due to the fact that we have little control over random stressful events that cause an emotional rollercoaster in our thought processes. That is why the next step of a strict ketogenic diet is needed for peri-menopausal and menopausal women to be able to lose weight. A standard ketogenic diet will aid all PMS and menopausal symptoms, but is often still not efficient enough for stubborn fat loss for women in this age group from my experience and I will explain why coming up.

The benefits of a ketogenic diet are many. Unfortunately, ketosis is sometimes confused with ketoacidosis, which is a rare condition that some diabetics can encounter which can be quite serious. Up until the 1920s, ketogenic diets were used to treat many disease processes in the body including diabetes, obesity, tremors, seizures, anxiety, bipolar disorder, schizophrenia and other forms of mental illness. Also, improvements in Alzheimer's disease, Parkinson's disease, epilepsy, and traumatic brain injury had been noted in certain studies. Ketogenic diets have also been studied for their neuro-protective effect which translates to a decrease in neuroinflammation resulting in a decrease in brain cell death. This is thought to be due to this more readily available fuel (ketones) for brain cells, which improves the brain cells' ability to resist negative metabolic changes. This concept is quite interesting when you contrast it with the fact that alcohol (the simplest form of a sugar/ carbohydrate) has been noted to kill brain cells. The brain can easily use a ketogenic diet for fuel because its ketone bodies can readily cross the blood brain barrier often by simple diffusion.

People will experience physical changes with the ketogenic diet such as deeper sleep, clearer thinking, improved digestion, increased energy, and less joint stiffness and pain. There are also changes that can be traced on medical tests such as lower blood pressure, decreases in overall cholesterol, increases in HDL, dropping triglycerides, as well as a drop in fasting blood sugar and fasting insulin levels.

The latest scientific studies have shown that a ketogenic plan is not detrimental to health if you do it while minimizing carbohydrate intake, which is obviously the point. If carbohydrates are not minimized, the body will burn the carbohydrates as fuel, and not the fat. A fairly recent study shows than normal low carbohydrate diet (ketogenic diet) versus a low-fat diet (which is higher in carbohydrates) proved better participant retention and greater weight loss and in addition to this, triglyceride levels decreased more and high density lipoprotein cholesterol levels increased more in the low carbohydrate diet.

Optimally, you should eat a diet with moderate protein, high in actual fats, and low in carbohydrates for the above listed benefits. Beware though that when you combine a lot of fat with a lot of carbohydrates, the sugar from the carbohydrates will increase your insulin levels, and then the high insulin levels cause all the carbohydrates that you eat to be stored immediately. This will obviously cause rapid weight gain and is associated with "insulin resistance" and the normal health problems associated with a high carbohydrate diet.

The more complex issue is that for women, typically those over thirty five, using this typical ketogenic diet, like the Atkins diet, no longer seems to work efficiently for fat loss. These types of ketogenic diets will; however, definitely aid in blood sugar balancing and mood stabilization, sleep improvement, and aid in lowering cortisol levels. This will allow a better balance between estrogen and progesterone, which results in a decrease in capable PMS and menopausal symptoms. So when the typical ketogenic diet no longer works, the only conclusion is for these women is to be forced to burn their own body fat by eating a low enough calorie diet so that the body registers a form of starvation, in order to warrant "going in and getting" these stubborn fat stores. This cannot be done with the present state of the hypothalamus, or many women would be successful by simply just starving themselves to lose body fat, which is not the case, nor is this healthy. There needs to be an impetus to balance the whole hormonal system or what I call a stimulus to cause the hypothalamus to stimulate these stubborn fat reserves to be released into the bloodstream. Again, this was a very natural state that we have veered away from in our modern society due to chronic stress and abuse of sugar/alcohol/caffeine. It is essential that we get back to this natural ketogenic, or fat burning, state especially as we age or weight (fat) loss will be impossible.

Dr. Simeon came up with a solution; his impetus to aid this process and aid the hypothalamus was hCG, the "pregnancy" hormone. This hormone, amongst other roles, stimulates the brain to release excess or abnormal fat around the stomach, hips, and thighs into the bloodstream when there are not enough calories for the woman (or her unborn baby) to survive. Dr. Simeons brilliantly translated this concept to men and women who needed to lose weight, and came out with a specific diet and protocol for the use of hCG. Within the last decade, hCG came out in a homeopathic form which made it very convenient for people to use in a safe and effective manner. The original version of my book in Chapter 3 went into this in great detail, and also detailed the media's issue with the use of hCG. I specifically wrote a rebuttal for each point in a very logical way. It is beyond the scope of this chapter to go into all of that in detail, so I will simply say that we used hCG in a homeopathic form successfully in my center for four years, until the FDA deemed it illegal to manufacture.

I understood this decision to be based on two basic reasons. The reasons did not deal specifically with safety, as there were no reported fatalities, injuries, issues with the use of hCG.

The FTC got involved due to "unsubstantiated claims" that dealt with companies who's advertising claimed that outrageous amounts of weight could be lost through the use of hCG and Dr. Simeon's 500 calorie diet protocol. It may have seemed that way, but I can tell you from experience, women would lose an average of twenty pounds per month and men could lose an average of thirty pounds per month. The other reason hCG was pulled of the market was the fact that hCG is not listed as one of the "grandfathered in" ingredients by the FDA in the Homeopathic Pharmacopeia. The Homeopathic Pharmacopeia has about 200 ingredients listed in it that were allowed to be made into homeopathic form when our country started and the AMA (American Medical Association) was formed. As a side note, any drug or herb can be made into a homeopathic solution, this just means that the drug or herb is diluted down, losing its potential side effects, but is still effective in gently nudging it in the direction it needs to go toward balance and health. Again, it is beyond the scope of this chapter to speak in depth about homeopathic medicine, except to say that it does not have the traditional side effects of allopathic medicines. See Appendix G for more in-depth information on homeopathic medicine.

Our success in my local BeBalanced center with the use of hCG (blended with other homeopathic ingredients) when included with a hormone balancing diet as part of our patent pending lifestyle-change protocol (as described in Chapter 8), was phenomenal, and was the reason I decided to write this book. Not only did women lose weight, but they were rid of many pesky PMS and menopausal symptoms, and had balanced hormones that could aid in the prevention of female related cancers, as well as rapid aging and the diseases/cosmetic issues that go with it.

With knowledge that hCG was soon going to be off the market, we began to do research on other ways to stimulate the hypothalamus to be able to function more normally, and to reset the metabolism back to normal, allowing for efficient weight loss. There still needed to be an impetus of a low-calorie diet, because if adequate calories were taken in, the body would always default to using those calories to survive, and would never use stored body fat which is always saved for a "famine."

That is where our attention turned to glandular therapy. Glandular therapies involve utilizing glands, organs, or tissue from healthy animals to improve the function of the same glands/organs in the patient or client. From a holistic perspective, this type of therapy is highly recommended over standard synthetic medications, due to the fact that these substances contain enzymes and cofactors that are used to support balance in the body, and there are no side effects when used properly.

Glandular tissue extracts come in pill form or homeopathic form for all of the major glands of the body such as the hypothalamus, pituitary, adrenal, ovarian, as well as the most widely used gland today, the thyroid gland. In recent years, more holistic practitioners have turned to glandular therapy and whole tissue supplementation in degenerative disorders and even immune mediated conditions that are often difficult to manage with traditional or conventional therapies.

To dispel any skepticism that this theory of taking glandulars will aid your glands, studies have been done where radioactive dyes have been used to demonstrate that large hormones, enzymes, proteins and peptides from a glandular supplement are routinely absorbed intact or only partially degraded, and that these constituents can concentrate in target tissues. These laboratory studies also document a more rapid uptake of the tagged cells (glandulars)or their components by traumatized organs over normal, healthy organs, leading to faster healing rates. This simply means that the glandular type that you take will have an affinity for (or attraction to) your matching gland in the body and the glandular will head right there to help repair that gland.

Because the most commonly used animal glandular is porcine (pig) thyroid gland called Armour Thyroid, and because this has been used for decades, it is a good example to point to for the common as well as safe use of animal glandular therapy. Armour Thyroid was the most popular treatment for hypothyroidism, up until the development of more synthetic form such as Synthroid which seems to have taken over the market. The debate as to which is better, synthetic or natural goes on but it should be noted that Armour Thyroid is much more natural to the body and contains T3 and T4. Unfortunately, with either medication it may be hard to get stable, consistent blood work results, due to thyroid conditions only being the result of major imbalances between sex and stress hormones (more on this in Chapter 4).

The first successful insulin preparations also came from cows, and then later from pigs. The insulin protein contained within the pancreas was isolated from pigs slaughtered for food, and then was purified, bottled, and sold. Later, a less expensive way to produce insulin was in the lab called "recombinant DNA" technology, and is now used for almost all insulin production.

The medical community has been trying to work with the thyroid and/or the pancreas as the two main glands zeroed in on to control blood sugar and weight, ignoring the full orchestra of hormones controlled by the hypothalamus. Neither of these drug applications (thyroid meds or insulin) will actually support the gland, but will simply take over and fill in the hormone in the body when the gland is not producing it. This will not aid the overall health of the body nor cause weight loss, the glands need to be supported and healed to restore balance in the body. I've never seen someone go on insulin or thyroid medication and lose weight as a result.

We need to think outside the box and look higher—literally higher, to the brain, and how the hypothalamus/pituitary connection specifically affects the supporting glands of the body (adrenal, thyroid, and pancreas glands) in order to have efficient fat loss. All of these glands need to be supported for the metabolism to be reset to normal via the hypothalamus, orchestrating the hormones as it was originally supposed to by the body. When this happens, hyper glands (ones under stress trying to overproduce hormone to keep up) can relax and rest and hypo glands (ones that have become exhausted and now produce less hormones) can come back into balance and heal, to produce the hormones what they were intended to produce. Again, as stated above, there needs to be an impetus to balance the whole hormonal system and a stimulus to cause the hypothalamus to release stubborn fat reserves into the bloodstream. Without the ability to use hCG to do this, due to it being unavailable, glandulars could be the next best viable option!

There are companies that successfully use glandulars in a safe and effective way. We chose to work with one that is known for the purity of their glandulars for over 30 years. What impressed me most about this company is the purity of their glandulars. They attain their glands and tissues from range-fed livestock that is not exposed to things like herbicides and pesticides, synthetic fertilizers, or growth hormones due to coming from New Zealand. The use of growth hormones is illegal in New Zealand and this is monitored very closely. It is also illegal in

New Zealand to send dirty livestock to packing plants. Animals are washed and inspected pre and post mortem - if there's a problem with the carcass of the animal, or any of the origins, both are destroyed in this type of rigorous inspection. This is not the case in Great Britain, Europe, or Canada where animals have been exposed to BSE, which is also known as Mad Cow Disease.

We began working with this company a few years back when we were introduced to one of their homeopathic glandular blends that was specifically made to replace hCG, and to aid the body in weight loss in a similar way. I prefer the homeopathic form of glandular therapy, because it is easy to use and there is no chance of overdosing. This blend, amongst other things, contains the hypothalamus, thyroid, adrenal, and pituitary glandulars in a safe homeopathic form. Like hCG, when used with a lower calorie diet of a specific ratio of carbohydrates to protein, the body will release stored body fat into the bloodstream to be used as the primary source of fuel, which is the definition of a state of ketosis. There was even an independently published study comparing pure homeopathic hCG to this homeopathic glandular formula showing similar results . This is the type of glandular therapy that we decided to switch to when homeopathic hCG was frowned upon by the FDA. We used their base formula that was proven effective in the study, and added some additional key homeopathic ingredients that were very successful in our original hCG blend. Then we also added homeopathic progesterone to further facilitate the balancing of estrogen and progesterone. This was then combined with our special lower calorie hormone balancing diet of lean meat, eggs, and low glycemic fruits and vegetables in an important 1 to 1 ratio of protein to carbohydrates.

Homeopathic glandular therapy combined with natural progesterone, like hCG, will support the orchestration of the glands in the body to easily allow a person to get into a ketogenic state when used with a lower calorie diet consisting of half protein and half low glycemic carbohydrates. The body can then use its own stored fat as the primary source of fuel, as opposed to a normal ketogenic diet in which high levels of fat are ingested and partially used as the main source of fuel along with body fat, so less fat is burned per day. A ketogenic state attained with the use of hCG or glandulars, however, will surprisingly not produce ketones in the urine, because the ketone bodies (fat) are being used as quickly as they are being produced. This is the most effective and efficient type of ketogenic diet, and the only choice for women who have tried every other type a diet with no results.

This is usually the only solution for peri-menopausal/menopausal women who cannot lose body fat from a regular low- calorie diet or a standard ketogenic diet such as the Atkins diet. The benefits of any ketogenic diet are long as stated above, but when the body's own abnormal fat stores are able to be used rapidly for fuel, weight loss can be fast as well as safe because the body will not use muscle (no catabolic effect of breaking down muscle). A person's blood sugar rapidly stabilizes and the body becomes more sensitive to insulin, the thyroid gland is no longer heavily taxed, and the adrenal gland has a chance to regenerate, while progesterone levels are able to rise to balance with estrogen. The results are not only rapid fat loss in areas where the woman has the most stored body fat (stomach, hips and thighs) but also improved mood/mood stabilization, improved sleep, and a rapid decrease in virtually all PMS and menopausal symptoms. Women will also notice a slow reversing in more serious female health issues such as fibroids, fibrocystic breasts, endometriosis or heavy menstrual cycles.

It may seem extreme by conventional diet standards but a protocol using a low calorie ketogenic diet (with a ratio of 1 to 1 of carbohydrates to protein) coupled with a safe homeopathic glandular blend , in all my experience, is needed for efficient fat loss for many peri and post menopausal women. It is the key combination of balanced blood sugar/ insulin of the ketogenic state, combined with the impetus of the glandulars to support the hypothalamus to be able to release stubborn, stored fat while rebalancing the orchestration of the other hormones in the body. This also takes extreme physiological stress off the body (aiding and rebuilding the adrenal gland), and although psychological stress needs to be monitored, the calming ketogenic state actually allows women to handle emotional stress better, becoming less likely to overreact, which often causes more emotional stress. Once balance is achieved and excess fat is lost, the woman becomes more sensitive to insulin, and can easily maintain balance with the support of natural hormone balancing creams. Supplementation with some natural progesterone will then maintain optimal levels to aid a woman psychologically (calmer mood, deeper sleep and less sugar cravings) and physiologically (less fat gain, better thyroid function and more energy for exercise). This is true natural hormone balancing. Then a woman will look and feel her best and can live each day to the fullest without constantly worrying and thinking, "How am I ever going to lose this excess weight?" There is such a freedom in that which allows her to live a much higher quality of life by pursuing her passion and following her dreams!

CHAPTER 4

The Hormone Shift & Thyroid

The Use of Thyroid Medication to Treat Symptoms . . .

What is typically the main cause of a woman's thyroid problems?
Why are so many women put on thyroid medication?
Why does conventional thyroid medication not ease all hormonal symptoms?
Solution: Balance hormones naturally and make lifestyle changes to correct thyroid issues.
Specifics on a natural hormone balancing solution (refer to Chapter 8)

O ver the years, I have heard many women say, "My blood tests show that my thyroid hormone is low, but taking Synthroid doesn't seem to alleviate my symptoms of weight gain, chronic fatigue, low libido, and thinning hair." This is often the case for women who take thyroid medication because of the indication of low levels of T4 on their standard thyroid test. Other factors contribute to this lack of relief, but the main cause is the hormonal shift of female sex hormones due to stress. The widely-used medical solution of solely supplementing with T4, will not fix the key underlying hormonal problem.

There also seems to be an increase in women who suspect that they may have a thyroid condition because they are displaying symptoms such as weight gain, chronic fatigue, low libido, and thinning hair. Often, their doctors disagree because their blood test results show that the thyroid hormone, thyroxine (T4), and the thyroid-stimulating hormone (TSH) levels both fall within the normal test range. So, why do these women continue to insist that there is something wrong? They do so based on intuition, which is an inner voice that says, "Something is off. I am gaining weight, losing hair, have no energy or sex drive, and

I can't think clearly!" This voice is right, something has shift ed! This is the beginning of a thyroid problem and when it is left unchecked, it can eventually lead to low T4 and elevated TSH. There is a root cause that needs to be addressed in order to avoid medication.

Sex and Stress Hormones Affect Your Thyroid

Stress, of course, is the preliminary culprit that starts the downward spiral of the thyroid gland. The constant "fight-or-flight" mode in which we live causes a hyper state of the thyroid well before the thyroid would be considered hypo (low). However, we rarely pay attention to the beginning stages because of our stressful lifestyles. In this period, we are functioning in the sympathetic (fight-or-flight) nervous system and it begins to take a toll on the body as the demand for cortisol rises. This demand, as stated in Chapter 1, will lower progesterone levels, shift ing you into a state of "estrogen dominance." Over time, this imbalance will negatively affect the thyroid gland because the excess estrogen "blocks" the thyroid hormones from working efficiently. Progesterone, known to support the thyroid gland, being low at this point will further complicate matters. Additionally, the excess cortisol that is produced (from converting progesterone to cortisol) can block the receptor sites of the thyroid hormone. Hormones need to hit their receptor sites in order to communicate with the cells. This series of events explains why your T4 (T3 is rarely tested) can show to be at an acceptable level and your TSH in the proper range on a standard thyroid test, but your thyroid gland is still not able to perform efficiently. What your doctor cannot observe from this test is that your thyroid hormones (T3 and T4) are being blocked by estrogen and cortisol. This common scenario will then allow your normal PMS symptoms to couple with additional hypothyroid symptoms (fatigue, cold extremities, hair loss, weight gain) beginning a further downward spiral. Furthermore, the neuro-chemical imbalances, which can coincide with the stress cycle, are connected with thyroid issues as well. Anxiety and depression will usually be a result of this as well (Read more in Chapter 6).

When you initially ask for a thyroid test based on the hypothyroid symptoms you are experiencing, your TSH and T4 levels will often show to be in acceptable ranges. This can be confusing to both you and your doctor. However, if your female hormone imbalance is left unchecked; over time, the thyroid gland will get lazy and produce less of the necessary thyroid hormone (Lee, 2004, p.224). The feedback system meant to maintain adequate thyroid hormone levels will eventually break down and T4 will appear low on a blood test. Subsequently, TSH levels rise as they work to push your body to produce more thyroid hormone. If your doctor was previously unconcerned, at this point you will finally have his/ her attention . . . a little too late!

From the very onset of the sex and stress hormone imbalance, the thyroid and its intended hormonal effect get weaker. Your energy levels have been vastly effected and this is usually the last straw, causing you—like so many women—to seek medical attention. At this point, a doctor may now decide to use a T4 medication (such as Synthroid) because of the displayed low energy levels combined with unacceptable ranges of T4 on blood tests. Then, the unthinkable happens—you are told that you need to be on T4 for the remainder of your life. And guess what? If you do not do anything to support your thyroid (by fixing your sex and stress hormone imbalance), your doctor is probably right.

Keys to Balancing Your Thyroid

The best solution for balancing your thyroid is to shift your female hormones (estrogen and progesterone) back into balance and get your stress hormones (mainly cortisol) under control. This will allow your thyroid gland to begin working as it should. In Chapter 8, I describe two very specific methods that will make this accomplishment possible. Both methods are natural and extremely effective. In this chapter, however, I will discuss some general lifestyle changes that will enable you to have a healthier thyroid gland. This will be followed by a discussion on how to potentially treat an already existing thyroid hormone imbalance with or without medication.

To confirm your sex hormone imbalance, which is the key to your thyroid issues, I suggest you answer a simple symptom-based hormone questionnaire. This will indicate a presence of low progesterone and "estrogen dominance" connected to adrenal fatigue/exhaustion (see the end of Chapter 1). Obviously, I cannot request that you move to a deserted island free of your children, husband, demanding boss, and job;

but I can suggest some simple lifestyle and diet changes, in combination with addressing your low progesterone and adrenal fatigue/exhaustion. It is important to note that high levels of stress hormones are associated with speeding up the aging process, while proper levels of balanced sex hormones are very anti-aging in nature. When balanced, your body will begin to think it is young and can still reproduce. I have seen many clients eliminate or lower thyroid medication with their doctors' assistance simply from balancing their sex and stress hormones.

Additional Suggestions to Support Your Thyroid Gland

I would like to go over some modifications you can make in your diet and lifestyle so that you may help to support your thyroid gland. The first thing is to be sure to eat plenty of protein. Women tend to favor carbohydrates over protein because they taste good, they are quick and easy, and they feed an emotional craving that seemingly nurtures us. However, eggs and poultry—especially turkey—are easy to digest and good for every blood type. Red meat can be enjoyed on occasion but it tends to be harder to digest; especially if you are an A blood type. Seeds and nuts are also a good option and they are easier to digest if you soak them in water overnight (releases their natural enzyme-inhibitors). If you are on-the-go, then a good protein drink would be fast and easy to digest. Rice protein, although not as well-known, is gentle on the digestive system. Additionally, there are also egg or whey protein drinks, but avoid soy protein for now (see below).

Protein aids in (1) balancing blood sugar, which lowers physical stress and calms us, (2) building lean body tissue and muscle with resistance training, and (3) providing all of the amino acids, which are the building blocks needed for growth, maintenance, and repair of the body. Amino acids (the building blocks of protein) are needed to make certain neuro- chemicals in the brain that affect our mood and behavior. There seems to be a direct connection between depression and low thyroid (hypothyroidism), and it is affected by the underlying hormonal imbalance that we just discussed. From what I have seen and understand, the connection might very well be that when we lack protein, or the enzymes to break it down, we are then low in amino acids such as L -tyrosine. L-tyrosine is needed to make thyroid hormones;

therefore, there is definitely some sort of hindrance in bodily function when we become protein deficient.

Protein consumption needs to be taken one step further. You can eat all of the protein in the world, but if it is not being digested properly, it will cause digestion and elimination problems. I suggest that my clients consume more protein and take a "professionally formulated" digestive enzyme; preferably, one that works in the stomach and upper intestine. This is referred to as a "dual-phase enzyme" and it is more effective. You can buy digestive enzymes at health food stores but they may not be as effective due to the lower concentrations of enzymes and they usually only work in the stomach. Digestive enzymes allow protein to be easily broken down into useful amino acids. Another factor to note is that after the age of twenty-five (which is not that old!) we lose our ability to break down protein adequately. These amino acids are more important than ever because of the excessively stressful lifestyles that we lead. The more stress that our bodies are under, the more they need to produce the stress hormone, cortisol. These stressors also require that our brain produces the neuro-chemicals (adrenaline and norepinephrine) as well. These neuro- chemicals aid in the initial fight-or-flight response and are made directly from the neuro-chemical, dopamine (the "happy" neuro-chemical). So, if the stress response is using up your dopamine to make adrenaline and norepinephrine for survival purposes, you will be apt to need more amino acids such as L-tyrosine. If dopamine levels continue to go down you will feel stressed, then drained, and eventually depressed. The lack of the amino acid L-tyrosine, which is needed to make thyroid hormones, will negatively affect your mood and your thyroid gland. I also suggest working under a health care professional when supplementing with L-tyrosine in order to support the thyroid gland—especially if depression is present. You can read more about neuro-chemicals, hormones and mood in Chapter 6.

To assist the thyroid in working properly, it is best to avoid certain foods or types of foods:

- **Peanuts and peanut butter** can block iodine usage in the body, which can affect production of the thyroid hormones. Try cutting these out for a time and substitute other nuts like almonds and cashews or the nut butters made from these nuts, in lieu of peanut butter.

- **Avoid soy for the same reason.** If you do consume soy products, make sure they are non-GMO (genetically modified). Also, be sure that you do not have a slight soy allergy or sensitivity. You can test your pulse five to ten minutes after eating a food to see if you are sensitive to it. Be sure to stay seated so you do not raise your pulse through activity. If pulse goes up ten or more beats per minute, your body is reacting and "not liking" that food. It should be avoided or eaten in small amounts or at least eaten with a digestive enzyme to help break it down.

- **Replace unsaturated oils (like corn, soybean, and other vegetable oils and margarine) that you may consume daily with the healthier alternatives such as coconut oil.** Coconut oil is more stable and is more easily broken down by the liver than the above listed unsaturated oils we normally consume. It also does not drain important metabolic enzymes the body needs for all metabolic processes. This is important due to the fact that the T4 thyroid hormone is converted by metabolic enzymes into the more active T3 thyroid hormone. Thus, preventing enzyme drainage, allowing these essential enzymes to be available for that conversion.

- **Avoid chemicals like sodium benzoate, potassium benzoate, aspartame, and saccharin found in almost all regular and diet sodas.** At a cellular level, almost all chemicals that are unnatural to the body will disrupt or impede what the thyroid hormone is trying to do in the cell, which is to produce energy!

Take Stress into Consideration

Americans are literally in fight-or-flight mode for most of the day. We need to break this daily stress pattern. Obviously, you cannot get rid of all of your stressors. The best way to break the daily stress pattern is to evoke the "relaxation response" for about twenty minutes every day. It offsets the stress response that engages the sympathetic nervous system. This stress response drains our hormones, nutrients, and neuro-chemicals. One of my favorite books on this subject is Dr. Herbert Benson's, *The Relaxation Response,* and it works! Think of it this way . . . after we sit at a desk all day, thirty minutes of physical activity at the gym helps to offset our sedentary lifestyle. The same thing happens with the brain—deep relaxation that evokes slowed brainwave patterns of alpha, theta, or even delta (deep healing can occur here) will offset the high gamma and beta brainwave patterns we experience all day. This can be accomplished through massage, meditation, and yoga. A realistic suggestion for busy women is to listen to a relaxation CD daily that uses "sound-wave" therapy with underlying relaxing music. In twenty or twenty-five minutes, you can feel like a new woman or one who just had a two-hour nap. Taking time for self-care demonstrates self-love in a practical way. In my center, we feel that "sound-wave" therapy is so important and we incorporate it into our full hormonal weight-loss program (details on our program in Chapter 8). On the Internet, research the words "sound-wave therapy" and you can find lots of CD options, or check out the work of Kelly Howell with the company, Brain Sync (see references). As with any "sound-wave" therapy, it is essential to use headphones to produce the full effect. This quiet "me time" can later be used for structured prayer time or a time of creative visualization of what you want your life to look like. This is especially helpful if you are not happy with your job, relationship, etc. Albert Einstein said, "Imagination is everything. It is the preview of life's coming attractions." Relaxation therapy is important because the subconscious mind is more receptive to the desires we may have when we are fully relaxed. This tool can be used to lower stress and to assist our lives to move more in the direction of our goals!

Emotions and the Thyroid Gland

Now, I would like to share with you a final thought in regard to the thyroid gland; there is usually an emotional component related to most thyroid conditions. This relates to both hyper and hypothyroidism. Eastern medicine adheres to the idea that all diseases have an emotional and a physical component and many times these are so fully intertwined that we can only see the physical symptoms. If a mental stress factor (say it is your job or marriage) is causing you to constantly think negative and stressful thoughts, then it is this "emotional issue" that causes your stress; and therefore, a need for increased cortisol production, which results in your subsequent low progesterone levels. This eventually affects the thyroid gland. Additionally, physical stressors like lack of sleep, too much sugar and too much caffeine, can stress the body as well. However, the strong emotional component is what leads us to this physical state and in turn creates the physical symptoms. It is doubtful that your doctor questions the state of your career or marriage when analyzing your T4 and TSH levels! So, let us touch on the "emotional component" here to see if this makes sense to you and then you can decide for yourself.

It is no secret that we, as women, like to talk and express ourselves; and if we do not feel like we are being heard, this can be extremely upsetting. When we cannot communicate correctly or as we would like to, we feel stifled. This happens in intimate relationships, with our teenage children, with our bosses, or even with some of our friends. This is partially due to the fact that, although liberated, we still live in a patriarchal society which can further add to that stifled feeling. When we feel suppressed, we do not want to "be a bitch" or be "unladylike," so we hold our tongue and suppress our feelings. However, our words are expressions of how we feel and an energy form that needs to be communicated (released) or this energy can build up in an unhealthy way. As discussed, stress affects our cortisol and hormone levels and ultimately affects the "chemistry" of our bodies. Furthermore, the buildup of suppressed emotions, over time, can adversely affect the "physics" of our body. Physics, the study of energy, is often ignored by the medical community in relation to our overall health. I strongly believe that this is an unaddressed "missing link" in our overall healing. Energy healing has only more recently become an accepted form of healing in the United States, but it still has far to go before most people generally accept it. It is, however, based on a valid science and has been used for thousands of years prior to allopathic medicine. Some common modalities that utilize energetic healing are homeopathic medicine (see Appendix G), Reiki, and acupuncture (now being accepted by insurance companies and doctors). The "physics" of your body can now be scientifically validated with a machine that will measure your individual energy level via a scale which measures hertz levels. This machine was made by Bruce Tainio of Tainio Technologies (an independent division of Eastern Stare University in Cheny, Washington). This machine was initially used to test the energies of soil, water and plants; but eventually, it was used in conjunction with the work of Dr. Gary Young to determine human frequency levels. Healthy human energy levels should be between 62-68 Hz. However, levels that fall far below this can be linked to all sorts of diseases, from common colds to cancer.

Let me now take this energy concept and apply it to your thyroid function. Eastern medicine supports the concept that there are energy centers, or vortexes, in all areas of the body known as chakras (meaning spinning wheels). Each chakra is associated with physical organs and emotional components. The one that specifically affects the thyroid gland is known as the throat chakra. Therefore, the throat chakra is physically associated with the thyroid, but emotionally it is connected to communication. The concept of chakras originated in the spiritual teachings of Hinduism and Buddhism but does not necessarily have ties to any one religious belief. It is scientific fact that our thoughts affect our bodies; there is a definite connection between our physical and emotional selves. Feeling stifled lowers the energy in the throat chakra and *will* affect your thyroid gland, just like the lack of energy flow to any other body part will affect its performance. It is theorized that blocked energy first starts in a gaseous nature but if not released it will form into liquid (causing thyroid cysts—often benign) and then later can form a solid mass if not released (causing thyroid nodules). Cancerous masses on the thyroid become present when there are other genetic and toxic factors as well. Medical science has no one theory on the direct underlying cause of thyroid issues, but energy science can make sense of this and it is directly tied to your emotions, which are intangible energies. Tying this together, it would make sense that the origin of the word, disease, stems from "dis"- ease (the lack of ease); which means you are existing in a stressful state.

I often suggest Reiki sessions to my clients to deal with emotional blockages in the throat chakra. Similar to acupuncture, Reiki channels positive energy to an area of the body where the energy is blocked or stifled. It is less expensive than acupuncture and noninvasive. If you doubt the power of human touch, then think of why it feels so good for you to hold your aching stomach with your hand, or why touching your child's fevered head or sore tummy brings relief. You do not need to be a physicist to understand this. Reiki is a relaxing therapy that allows for the release of pent-up emotions from differing areas of the body. It is a form of energy medicine, and I assure you, it is based on the science of energy. Some hospitals even allow nurses to use it, as it is soothing, safe, and noninvasive. Additionally, using a "sound-wave" therapy CD, paired with a mental exercise (see the *Lighten Up Emotionally* exercise in Appendix A), will allow you to release your emotions very effectively as well.

You may be asking yourself, "How does the physical-emotional connection apply to me?" Take a look at your life and analyze what is going on—now or in the recent past. Were you always able to fully communicate with your spouse, your teenager, or your boss? Do you feel like you had something to say but could not say it because you did not want to cause an argument, get fired, or hurt someone's feelings? We all suppress some of our emotions, and it is certainly a good thing to not always blurt out what is on our mind, but chronically suppressing our emotions can be extremely problematic. The answers to these questions can help you better understand the emotional component of your thyroid issue. This kind of inner work is hard; anything emotional is often hard to deal with. However, you will grow from this, be a better person, and a better example to others around you. Try communicating with love to the person with whom you have the issue. You are not saying you are right and that he or she is wrong. You are just communicating how you feel and it is always good to be able to validate your feelings by expressing them. Determine if the issue is really worth pursuing, and if it is, maybe call the person or send a heart-felt e-mail or letter expressing your thoughts. If the issue is not worth pursuing, then maybe just let it go, which is always an option if you can actually let it go. Perhaps, talk about it with a friend or therapist if you cannot talk to the person directly. If this person is just a friend, you may find you do not need to be with them as often. If this person is your spouse or a family member, it would do you good to try to work on communicating clearly. Remember, it will probably make them feel better in the process as they may really desire to know what issue is bothering you.

Ultimately, getting your sex and stress hormones balanced, making some simple diet modifications, taking stress management into consideration, and looking deeper at the emotional root of your thyroid issue will all positively affect your thyroid gland. You will end up feeling more energetic while allowing your body to rebalance itself and work more efficiently.

When Already taking Thyroid Medication

If you have already been diagnosed with a hypothyroid and your T4 levels are low, packing in synthetic T4, such as Synthroid, or other thyroid medications is really not the best solution. Doing so will often cause the thyroid gland to become lazy, decreasing its production of natural T3 and T4. This will result in you having to depend on thyroid medication for the remainder of your life. Most people do not want to take medications but it is easier to listen to their doctor so they accept this route as the only solution. This may be a cultural and societal problem related to our attitude toward modern medicine. We seem to be learning the hard way that medication is only a bandage.

Medication causes more stress on your body by increasing toxicity and side effects, plus the medications do not address all of your symptoms and never will. Most women that I see who are on synthetic thyroid medications—T4 alone, the common solution used by doctors—still have hair loss, foggy thinking, energy ups and downs, and weight issues. These symptoms will not dissipate until you balance your sex and stress hormones.

Furthermore, do drugs work for chronic issues? Sure they do, to some extent, or no one would use them. Taking a thyroid drug will acceptable range when measured on the standard medical test mentioned earlier. But as we discussed, this is not a true answer to the problem. In my twenty-three years of working in health and weight loss, I have never seen a woman lose weight after starting synthetic T4. Lack of synthetic T4 is not the problem—there is not a direct cause-and-effect relationship to weight issues. There are other hormonal imbalances that need to be addressed before weight can be lost efficiently. True balance only comes with lifestyle changes even after regularly taking a thyroid medication.

If you are already on thyroid medication, consider balancing your female hormones. Your thyroid hormones will then be able to work more efficiently and alleviate many stubborn symptoms that you are dealing with. Your thyroid hormone output will often become stronger and you may be able to lower your medication with your doctor's help.

If you desire to work with your doctor to convert to a more comprehensive and/or balanced approach to supporting your thyroid, below are some options you can share with him or her. It is vital for your doctor to cooperate by monitoring your TSH, T3, and T4 levels. If you do not monitor your levels carefully, there is danger of over-medication resulting in symptoms of hyperthyroidism, including heart palpitations, intolerance to heat, inability to sleep, and jittery feelings.

Three Options to Balance Your Thyroid

Here are a few examples to give you an idea of your options . . .

Option 1 (not highly recommended): Ask your doctor to add a prescription T3 drug (Cytomel, for example) to the already prescribed thyroid medication, which is often only T4 (Synthroid, for example). As stated earlier, T3 is the stronger and more active form of T4. T4 is converted into T3 so that the body may optimally function. It is essential for you to get rid of all of your symptoms, not just some of them. This method is a broader-spectrum application and will aid in dealing with more of your symptoms than T4 alone. Also, note that long-term use of T4 alone will tend to make the thyroid lazy and it will often not produce adequate thyroid hormones on its own. At this point you will be dependent on thyroid medication *unless* a natural supplement is used to support the thyroid. See the more "natural" ideas below.

Option 2: Cease taking your synthetic medication and replace it with a more effective supplement called a glandular. Glandulars are typically used to support various glands in the body and are made from the glands of animals. They contain all the enzymes and co-factors that the full spectrum naturally-produced hormone would. This makes them better recognized by the human body. Thyroid glandulars have trace levels of natural T4 and T3 *plus* the ability to be able to support the body with nutrients like selenium and L-tyrosine, which both allow the body to make its own thyroid hormones naturally. This method also has a tendency to keep the thyroid gland from getting lazy (which is caused by synthetic T4). This will possibly balance out the hypothalamus-pituitary-thyroid feedback loop (called HPT axis) which is the body's natural balancing system, utilizing TSH for overall balance.

An example of this type of formula offered by naturopathic doctors, or some doctors of osteopathic medicine (D.O.), may look something like this:

Vitamin A (as beta-carotene)
Vitamin B-2 (as riboflavin)
Calcium (as calcium citrate, calcium chelate)
Iodine (from Norwegian kelp)
Magnesium (as magnesium oxide)
Zinc (as zinc citrate, zinc chelate)
Manganese (as manganese citrate, manganese chelate)
Potassium (as gluconate)
Thyroid (freeze-dried)
L-Tyrosine
Proprietary Blend (freeze-dried adrenal, freeze-dried pituitary, freeze-dried spleen, freeze-dried thymus)
Irish moss seaweed (Chrondus crispus)
Parsley leaf (Petroselinum crispun)
Horsetail herb (Equisteum arvense)

This is an example of a blend that only professionals, like a medical doctor, osteopathic doctor, naturopathic doctor, chiropractor or other degreed and certified healthcare professionals may dispense. Used under their guidance it will allow you to totally eliminate thyroid medication (unless your thyroid gland has been removed) and will provide better broad spectrum results.

Option 3: If you are not fully comfortable with switching your synthetic medication to a glandular, there is another option to try. Augment your synthetic medication with a natural nutritional support for the thyroid gland, consisting of both iodine and iodide. The body can sometimes have a problem converting iodine to iodide. Iodide is essential to the production of thyroid hormones. It revitalizes the body and allows it to produce more of its own natural thyroid hormone. With your doctor's help in monitoring your hormone levels, the synthetic drug you are taking can probably be lowered over time. Other components, such as stress management and natural progesterone therapy, will be *key* to making this process much more effective. I suggest you work with a qualified health professional, although you can get this supplement online or at a health-food store. An example of this type of formula would be something like this:

Iodine—5 mg
Potassium Iodide—7.5 mg
Selenium—15 mcg
Vitamin B2 (Riboflavin)—15 mg L-tyrosine

In conclusion, there are many options you can try in order to take care of symptoms that you feel are directly or indirectly related to your thyroid gland. Your doctor may not give your symptoms credence until your thyroid issue is extremely problematic and you begin to display full- blown hypothyroidism, clinical depression, or female-related cancers. Why not catch these hormonal imbalances as soon as possible and rid yourself of the annoying symptoms that lower the quality of your life? You can look and feel better, as well as prevent long-term chances of deadly disease. For more information on specific ways to balance sex and stress hormones, see Chapter 8. If your thyroid issue causes you weight problems, see Chapter 3, or if your mood is greatly affected, see Chapter 6.

CHAPTER 5

The Hormone Shift & PMS

The Use of the Birth Control Pill to Treat Symptoms . . .

Why do women experience PMS symptoms?
Why is the Birth Control pill (BCP) being used for PMS symptoms?
How does the BCP work to ease PMS symptoms?
What affect does the BCP have on the body over a long period of time?
Solution: use natural hormone balancing to eradicate PMS symptoms
Specifics on a natural hormone balancing solution (refer to Chapter 8)

Almost all women and teenage girls seem to exhibit some sort of PMS (pre-menstrual syndrome) symptoms one to two weeks before the onset of their period. The shift of hormones that occurs at puberty, which naturally brings on menstruation, can be the start of these common discomforts; including mood swings, bloating, headaches, and food cravings followed by cramps, low energy and even an excessive menstrual flow. Stress of any kind can often be the cause of an imbalance between estrogen and progesterone, leading to many PMS symptoms even at the young age of puberty. You may be thinking, "What stress does a thirteen year old girl have that could deplete her progesterone levels causing symptoms of a hormonal imbalance? It is not like these young girls have taxes, jobs, husbands or children!" This is true, but remember from Chapter 1, that stress can also be from unknown food sensitivities, toxins in the body, lack of sleep, emotional issues from childhood or even inherited tendencies towards imbalances. These annoying and painful PMS symptoms have become so prominent that the medical community sought a more permanent solution than simply administering high levels of OTC drugs for pain (example, *Pamprin*). Over the past two to three decades, the birth control pill (BCP), which always was noted as relieving some of these PMS symptoms, has become the most commonly prescribed treatment for any girl who has even mildly symptomatic periods. It is even prescribed to young women who desire to skip the process of monthly menstruation altogether. The BCP is now being used outside of its primary role in pregnancy prevention to deal with slight to severe PMS symptoms.

You, like so many other women, may be starting to wonder, "Is long-term use of the birth control pill safe to prevent pregnancy, alleviate symptoms of PMS, and eliminate monthly periods?" The answer is that long-term use of the birth control pill has not yet been proven safe. The pill is nothing more than low-level synthetic hormones, of which the long- term use was proven unsafe in the 2002 *Women's Initiative Study*. This study, referred to in Chapter 2, shows that long-term use of *any* synthetic hormone can jeopardize the overall health of the endocrine system. The BCP has many major, as well as minor side effects. The benefits of the BCP will only temporarily mask hormonal imbalances and will also suppress natural hormone production, which can potentially cause more serious health-related problems over many years of use.

Since the introduction of the BCP, its use has grown tremendously beyond its obvious intended purpose. Therefore, a further discussion is warranted about how the BCP impacts your endocrine system. Many sub-clinical issues caused by its use can affect your body from the moment you take it as well as over time. Even if you do not display any of the labeled, rare and dangerous side effects while taking the BCP, you will want to make sure you are well educated in this subject matter.

In my heath center, approximately two -thirds of my clients who are taking the BCP are on it for reasons other than pregnancy prevention. Most of these reasons are for reducing PMS symptoms and for creating less frequent, lighter periods. While being able to outsmart Mother Nature seems like a great modern convenience, we need to ask ourselves, "Is this convenience worth the risk?" Also, we need to determine if the BCP is a viable symptom-control method that can be used safely through the teenage and adult years.

The BCP is comprised of synthetic hormones similarly to how synthetic HRT is composed of synthetic hormones. We know that most women have hormonal issues near menopause but even the average teenage girl has a hormonal shift each month after ovulation. This can make the last two weeks of her month (luteal phase) uncomfortable.

Therefore, the BCP is often prescribed to these girls just as synthetic HRT is prescribed to menopausal women for their symptoms. According to the FDA, however, any hormonal therapy should be used at the lowest effective dose that will treat your symptoms and for the shortest period of time. This does not seem to apply to the BCP from what can be observed. Doctors are now prescribing the BCP without an advisable end date. I have seen girls on the BCP until they are ready to start a family; oftentimes, from the ages of fourteen to thirty. It is no wonder that such a girl may have a troublesome time when they try to become pregnant!

The common side effects of the BCP are obvious but there are also rare, yet potentially life-threatening side effects as well. The problem is that most women (and I am guessing most young girls) assume that they are the exception to these extreme possibilities and most often, they are right. In this chapter, however, the sub-clinical issues (will not show up on lab tests) that the BCP brings about over time, will be discussed. Long-term overuse of this type of hormonal treatment erodes the body of its delicate hormonal balance. These imbalances can occur whether or not you ever display the "more serious" side effects that the drug companies are required to bring to your attention.

You may be asking, "If these synthetic hormone options are potentially dangerous, why do doctors continue to prescribe them?" There are a myriad of reasons! Hormonal imbalances have worsened as toxins in our food and environment have increased, nutrients in our soils have declined, and stressors in our modern society have multiplied. Our bodies struggle with all of these issues as we age, and synthetic hormones have become a go-to solution for controlling our problematic symptoms. In my professional opinion, this type of treatment should not be a treatment at all. Let us look at what these synthetic hormones are really doing to us, and then we will be able to see how naturally balancing our hormones can be just as effective in relieving symptoms without the potential dangerous side effects. This will allow you, as a conscious consumer, to make a genuinely informed choice.

How the Birth Control Pill Prevents Pregnancy

The main goal of the birth control pill is to prevent the reproductive system from releasing an egg; in other words, it suppresses ovulation. If an ovary does not release an egg, there is no way for a sperm to fertilize it. Another way the BCP prevents pregnancy is that it increases cervical mucus, causing it to become thick and tacky. This serves two purposes, sperm have a more difficult time getting through and the lining of the uterus becomes less receptive for implantation.

During the first half of a woman's cycle, called the "follicular phase," natural estrogen is produced in order to stimulate the follicles to form so that they can be used for fertilization. Estrogen is also used to stimulate the growth of the lining of the uterus, which makes a spot for the potentially fertilized follicle to implant. After ovulation, at which time a follicle matures and is released, the "corpus luteum" (the spot where the follicle was released) begins to produce progesterone. This is one of the main sources of progesterone for pre-menopausal women. During the second half of a woman's cycle, called the "luteal phase," natural progesterone continues to rise in order to prepare a woman's body for pregnancy. At the end of two weeks, if fertilization of the released follicle does not occur, a drop in progesterone causes the lining of the uterus to fall away, and this eventually causes menstruation.

The BCP contains high levels of synthetic estrogen. The use of it will throw off the feedback system that the hypothalamus relies on to signal the pituitary gland to start the process of stimulating a follicle for ovulation. If this natural balance or feedback system is thrown off, the hormonal sequence mentioned above does not occur and the body does not *really* produce any natural estrogen, or progesterone from the ovaries, and ovulation cannot occur; therefore, conception would not be possible.

The Basic Hormonal Imbalance in Women Today

The primary imbalance in women, which causes many uncomfortable hormone-related symptoms, is higher estrogen in relationship to progesterone; as mentioned in Chapter 1. This imbalance is the root of all PMS and menopausal symptoms, and relief from these symptoms has contributed to the increased use of synthetic hormones in the form of the BCP. The reason we currently have more PMS and severe menopausal symptoms is because of our elevated stress levels. The problem is that this is not temporary, but rather ongoing because we are under constant stress! This leaves us chronically low in progesterone, the hormone that helps us to maintain our weight, calms our mood, and keeps PMS symptoms away. In turn, we are left in an "estrogen dominant" state.

When the body is left with too much estrogen in relation to progesterone, all of the unwanted symptoms like headaches, irritability, mood swings, cramps, weight gain, depression, and anxiety become prominent. In older women, hot flashes and night sweats are added to the list. An even more serious problem is that too much estrogen can cause uncontrolled proliferation (growth) of the cells of the breast, uterus, ovaries, and cervix. This condition can set the stage for endometriosis, fibroids, cysts, and even female-related cancers as discussed in Chapter 2. You can see that this imbalance does not just inconvenience us with longer, heavier, more symptomatic periods, but can lead to serious conditions and diseases. This concept of "estrogen dominance" shows that the use of extra estrogen in a synthetic form, such as in the BCP, worsens the initial hormonal imbalance.

What really happens when we layer synthetic hormones on top of this imbalance of too much estrogen and not enough progesterone? The effect is complex to say the least, but some trends emerge from long-term usage of the BCP.

How Synthetic Hormones Cause Long-term Problems:

1. Synthetic hormones do not have all the necessary co-factors (enzymes) to do their job properly like natural hormones do. Example: Synthetic progesterone (called progestin) will regulate period like natural progesterone but will not aid in weight loss like real progesterone. Instead, it will actually cause fluid retention and weight gain!

2. Synthetic hormones will not be broken down by or respond to essential enzymes that render them inactive after they have done their job (telling a cell what to do), so they continue to over-stimulate cells in a dangerous way, possibly leading to cancers over time.

3. Synthetic hormones tend to cause "insulin resistance" (associated with elevated estrogen) which will always cause weight gain (especially around the midsection).

4. Synthetic hormones will kill intestinal flora (good bacteria) and allow for the overgrowth of Candida yeast. This will then cause the woman to crave sugar/starches, "bloat up" when she consumes sugar/starches; then over time, clog her system and cause weight gain. Also, low amounts of intestinal flora will lay the ground work for constipation as intestinal flora aids bowel transit time. Lymphatic movement will also tend to slow down causing the accumulation of toxins and fluid. If left unchecked for long periods of time, yeast turns into spores that bore into and perforate the intestinal wall. This process will allow food particles into the bloodstream, which causes an immune response and the creation of food sensitivities. These "sensitive" foods then become addicting, are often craved, and many times will contribute to weight gain (common examples: wheat and dairy).

5. Synthetic hormones increase the risk of birth defects, such as heart and limb defects, if taken during the first four months of pregnancy.

6. Synthetic hormones may contribute to thrombophlebitis, pulmonary embolism, and cerebral thrombosis.

7. Synthetic hormones may cause fluid retention, epilepsy, migraines, asthma, cardiac or renal dysfunction.

8. Synthetic hormones may cause breakthrough bleeding or menstrual irregularities.

9. Synthetic hormones may cause or contribute to depression due to excess estrogen and the increase in serotonin levels

Final warning: The effect of prolonged use of synthetic hormones on pituitary, ovarian, adrenal, hepatic, and uterine function is unknown.

Synthetic Estrogen in the BCP

Synthetic hormones in the BCP or HRT, no matter what the dosage, are drug-like in their effects. This means that they force the body in a certain direction and are not intended to create the true balance that the body needs. The synthetic estrogen used in the BCP is an imitation of natural estradiol (the most abundant estrogen in the body), and it is called ethinylestradiol.

This synthetic form of estrogen is made from the urine of animals like sheep, pigs, and horses. These are foreign estrogen molecules to the human body and do not have all the necessary co -factors (enzymes) to properly do their job like natural estrogen. This synthetic form of estrogen is often utilized because it can be patented by drug companies.

Our body's natural estrogen (estradiol) is also much weaker than the synthetic counterpart, ethinylestradiol. This synthetic version will suppress natural estrogen production from the ovaries and the adrenal gland, which are the main production sources. This can eventually decrease the protective effect that natural estrogen has on the heart. Ethinylestradiol is extremely potent, which will not allow the liver to break it down easily like natural estrogen. This fact causes synthetic estrogen to produce an additional surge in the body that hits cells a second time with its excitatory message. This leaves the door open for proliferation of the cells of the cervix, uterus, ovaries and breasts making cancer a more likely possibility. Synthetic hormones do not render inactive after they have hit their intended receptor sites (completing their job) due to the inability of the body to break them down with natural enzymes. Often, these synthetic hormones "overwork" in the body causing damage over time.

In contrast, natural hormones always have the necessary enzymes and co -factors to allow them to work safely and efficiently. The fact is that natural estrogen (mainly estradiol) is only produced three days out of a cycle and the liver can and does break it down to avoid overdosing on it. Natural hormones are further kept in balance by sex hormone binding globulin (SHBG), which keeps hormones such as estrogen from over- stimulating the body. I believe this safety measure was specifically put in place to keep balance in the body's hormone levels. SHBG works in tandem with the hypothalamus and pituitary feedback system that the body uses to orchestrate its hormones. However, synthetic ethinylestradiol in the BCP is not bound by SHBG and can easily get out of hand and surge to very high and dangerous levels.

As I have previously stated, if left unchecked without the balancing effect of natural progesterone, even natural estrogen will have a tendency to cause problems and symptoms. Ethinylestradiol, the man-made "monster" used in the BCP, is resistant to being broken down and can reach levels that are much more dangerous than natural estrogen. This is the very reason why the 2002 *Women's Initiative Study* on HRT was stopped; it was concluded that women were developing cancers due to increased levels of this synthetic hormone. Cancer may not statistically be a problem in young women, but synthetic hormones used at any time can lay the groundwork for cancer later in life. The ethinylestradiol found in the BCP might be less dangerous for younger women, but using the BCP for many years is likely throwing these young women's bodies off balance and setting them up for life-altering problems in the future.

Ethinylestradiol in the BCP is considered a xenoestrogen, which differs chemically from phytoestrogen (plant-estrogens) and natural estrogens produced by the body. This means xenoestrogen has a similar action (excitatory) as the hormone estrogen, but it is foreign to the human body. "Xeno," meaning "alien" or "strange," makes this type of estrogen more harmful than natural estrogen for men, women, and children. Xenoestrogens are considered harsh for the environment and are released into the water supply via the urine and feces of women on the BCP. This pollutes our water, mutates our fish, and is also linked to a rise in male infertility caused by drinking the tainted water. If this goes on, no one will ever have to worry about getting pregnant again because men will be sterile! How is that for irony and nature putting us in our place?

Another main source of xenoestrogens is plastics. Microwaving food in plastic containers is one way that xenoestrogens get into our food. Using glass containers is much safer and helps us avoid this additional source of estrogen. Many common water bottles contain a plastic polycarbonate that releases a chemical known as bisphenol A (BPA). When reviewed, a full 90% of governmental studies have found harmful health effects from BPA and its action as a xenoestrogen. BPA has also been linked to a higher incidence of breast cancer because it is "extra estrogen" coming into the body and we already have too much! Compounding this is the fact that BPA is in an unnatural toxic form.

We also consume xenoestrogens inadvertently through bottled water, which most of us drink to be healthier. Most bottled water is highly acidic and I have seen this demonstrated right in front of my eyes by a water representative from Kangen, a Japanese water ionization company. The representative tested all of the popular waters from Fiji to Smart Water, so that he could show me their acidity levels. Since popular waters sold to consumers are highly acidic, they will leech plastic from their bottles. Common plastic water bottles are another dangerous source of xenoestrogens. I have listed in the resources how you can find a machine to alkalize your water. This water comes conveniently from your own sink and eliminates the need to buy it in plastic bottles. This is just one way to lighten your load of extra estrogens in the body.

SIDENOTE: Not only will acidic water leech the plastic from the bottle in which it is stored and increase our levels of xenoextrogens, but it also leeches minerals out of bones. Calcium is used to nullify the effects of the body's overly acidic state which can contribute to osteoporosis as well. (This discussion is beyond the scope of this book but I want you to be aware of it).

Progestin in the BCP versus Natural Progesterone

The BCP does not use natural progesterone but rather a synthetic form of progesterone called progestin. Synthetic progestin comes in many forms (first, second, and third generations) that are lumped into a group called "progestins." These synthetic progestins used in the BCP are not the same as the progesterone your body produces naturally.

The synthetic progestin used in the BCP helps balance the synthetic estrogen in the BCP, but does not perform all of the positive functions that natural progesterone was meant to perform. Synthetic progestin will perform some of the same functions in the body as real progesterone such as regulating a period or reducing monthly menstrual cramps. However, the synthetic derivatives are not a substitution for real progesterone. Progestin does not have the protective effect against female-related cancers that natural progesterone does. This means that it does not lower the incidence of cancer when used with synthetic estrogen, especially if the synthetic estrogen prescribed causes long-term elevated levels in the bloodstream.

The double trouble caused by the BCP is that natural progesterone production will decrease in the body due to the cessation of ovulation and the inability of the corpus luteum (place where follicle is released) to produce it. In a young woman who is menstruating, the corpus luteum is the main source of natural progesterone in the body. Natural progesterone produced by the adrenal gland will almost always have been long taxed and depleted because of its quick conversion into cortisol (due to our stress-filled lives). Remember, natural progesterone is a key fat-burner and diuretic, will keep your weight in check, and aid in weight loss if needed. Progesterone also soothes the mood, aids in deeper sleep, and truly balances estrogen levels (both natural and synthetic forms) to aid in preventing female-related cancers. Use of the BCP diminishes our already lowered levels of this important sex hormone.

Where Do Synthetic Hormones Come From?

As stated above, synthetic estrogen (ethinylestradiol) is made from the urine of animals like sheep, pigs, and horses. Synthetic forms of progesterone (progestin) used in the BCP were discovered by the pharmaceutical companies while looking for a fertility drug as they were studying folk medicine in Mexico. Wild yams were found to have diosgenin, the base compound of progesterone. Diosgenin can easily be made into safe and natural progesterone. Some molecules are cleaved off of the diosgenin, with progesterone as the result. The problem is, real USP progesterone is like Vitamin C, it cannot be patented, so no real money can be made by drug companies. Therefore, conjugated artificial estrogens like ethinylestradiol (see previous section) and artificial progestins were invented and patented to protect market share. These artificial hormones can have serious side effects when used long term. Progestin is made by taking real progesterone and molecularly changing it so that it has some of the necessary effects of real progesterone but many negative side effects as well; just read the tiny print that comes with the BCP.

The pharmaceutical companies maintain large farms of yams to give them the base compounds for the manufacturing of their artificial hormones. Some of this crop is used in their production of bio-identical hormones as well, which tend to be structurally closer to what the body produces naturally. This type of bio -identical hormone therapy (discussed fully in Chapter 2) should not be confused with synthetic HRT or the synthetic hormones in the BCP.

It is interesting to note that all types of synthetic progestin have some estrogenic and androgenic effects instead of only progestational effects (see Appendix E for each example). Drug companies do admit to this and it is in the BCP literature. This point further emphasizes that only real (natural) progesterone will have all the valuable properties necessary in order to avoid PMS, menopausal symptoms, female-related cancer, and weight gain. You may be wondering, "Why on earth would anyone take a natural substance and make it synthetic in a process that takes time and costs money, when it is not nearly as safe or effective as the real substance?" The answer . . . Money. *It's that simple!* Unfortunately for drug companies, they cannot patent what is natural and no one seems to be able to improve on Mother Nature.

Birth control to avoid pregnancy is one case for which you may use the BCP besides aiding in PMS symptom control. Keep in mind that natural progesterone supplementation will also alleviate PMS symptoms, but it does not disrupt ovulation; therefore, will obviously not prevent pregnancy. However, also remember that natural progesterone will regulate your cycle so that your period comes with ease and predictability and you can use more of the rhythm or natural method to prevent pregnancy in lieu of the BCP. Nowadays, it seems that newer commercials and marketing are geared for women to use the BCP to skip periods out of convenience and to get relief from PMS and other symptoms. They even mention that the BCP aids in obtaining clearer skin. That is good marketing! Who really wants to get a period and who wants to be miserable when they get it? By appealing to young girls and women in this way, sales are dramatically increased even when the audience is not sexually active! The reason a period is such a "pain" to endure each month is because young girls and young women are hormonally imbalanced and must deal with lots of irritating symptoms. If natural progesterone is used, periods are regulated, come easily, are shorter, and are not such a big deal. Plus, with the use of natural progesterone, long-term health and anti-aging is enhanced and quality of life is increased.

It kills me when I hear this one commercial for a popular brand of a BCP. It advertises that you can get your period only four times a year, hooray! The annoying jingle starts off something like this, " Who says you have to get a monthly period? Who says you have to deal with it every month? Who says . . . Who says . . . ?" and I'm thinking, "I don't know, maybe God!" While the commercial seems to portray that there is no medical need for a period if you are not trying to conceive, I am also thinking, according to the medical community, there is no real medical need for a uterus as you age or ovaries either, so we can just remove them. There is also no medical need for breasts after childbirth either, which works out great because they may need to be removed anyway due to cancers brought on by the imbalance that these drugs may cause. It only makes sense that every organ in a woman's body is needed for balance and put there for a reason . . . Come on, *how dumb do they think the average woman is?*

Types of Synthetic Progesterone

All combination BCPs contain estrogen (typically ethinylestradiol) and one of the eight types of progestin. The term progestin, as stated above, is used for any natural or man-made substance that has some properties similar to natural progesterone. To best understand how a progestin may be classified, it is helpful to clarify the types of effects a progestin may have on the female body in terms of progestational, estrogenic, and androgenic activity. Also, progestins are categorized by generation. Try to locate your type of progestin for the type of BCP you are taking on this list located in Appendix E so you can learn of the effect it has on your body.

Due to the fact that progestin is slightly different on a molecular level from natural progesterone, there are specific side effects to each new form, or generation, that the drug companies create.

In review, remember that only natural progesterone is a fat-burner, a diuretic, and calming in nature which eases anxiety. Plus, it balances out "estrogen dominance" to protect against female-related cancers. Only real progesterone provides true "progestational" activity and binds to the necessary receptor sites. This beneficial activity balances out estrogenic and androgenic (male hormone) effects. You will see in Appendix E that all progestins do not provide purely "progestational" activity but rather have some estrogenic and androgenic affects, which can lead to imbalances and other problems, some not yet fully known or understood.

Appendix E clearly shows the breakdown of the three main generations of synthetic progestin, listing the positive effects as well as the specific negative effects for each generation. The third generation pills are a bit closer to natural progesterone; therefore, it does appear as if the pharmaceutical companies are trying to improve upon their formulations. If you must use the BCP for birth-control purposes, I would suggest this generation, but I also suggest that you work with a healthcare professional and combine it with additional natural topical progesterone cream to give your body some of the real, full advantages of progesterone. To my knowledge and through all of my experience, there has been no evidence that using natural progesterone in order to outweigh some of the risks of the BCP will deactivate the pill and cause increased risk of pregnancy. The benefits that I have seen when working with my clients are decreases in almost all PMS symptoms, weight loss, and improved mood by the lessening of depression and anxiety, better digestion and elimination, and eradication of Candida yeast overgrowth (find out more on natural progesterone in Chapter 8).

What Type of BCP are You on?

Monophasic birth control pills deliver the same amount of estrogen and progestin every day.

Biphasic birth control pills deliver the same amount of estrogen every day for the first 21 days of the cycle. During the first half of the cycle, the progestin/estrogen ratio is lower to allow the lining of the uterus (endometrium) to thicken as it normally does during the menstrual cycle. During the second half of the cycle, the progestin/ estrogen ratio is higher to allow the normal shedding of the lining of the uterus to occur.

Triphasic birth control pills have constant or changing estrogen concentrations and varying progestin concentrations throughout the cycle.

It is generally medically accepted that there is no evidence that biphasic or triphasic oral contraceptives are superior to monophasic oral contraceptives, or vice-versa, in the prevention of pregnancy.

What can be Done Naturally for PMS Symptoms?

Hormones can be balanced through the gentle and safe method of increasing progesterone levels as was mentioned in Chapter 1. The balance of hormones will aid in almost all PMS (and menopausal) symptoms dealing with mood, weight, and overall health. In this balanced state, you are in a much better position to be able to burn body fat, reduce fluid retention, and lower blood pressure and cholesterol. If you were taking the BCP for symptom control only (not contraception), you will find you no longer need to use it and you will avoid the long-term dangers.

What you need to consider in this process of choosing a specific form of natural progesterone therapy, as well as how to address your adrenal fatigue/exhaustion, will be discussed in Chapter 8. I have utilized this type of natural therapy for many years with great success with my younger, as well as my peri/postmenopausal clients.

Although rare, it is important to note here, that if progesterone levels are left too low (induced by stress) for too long, coupled with the long-term use of the BCP, natural estrogen's effectiveness can eventually be reduced and lead to some premature symptoms of menopause like hot flashes and night sweats when the BCP is stopped. This can even occur in young women after long-term use of the BCP! These symptoms can show up well before DHEA becomes low and estrogen also becomes low due to what was referred to as true "second-level" depletion mentioned in Chapter 1. Progesterone aids in estrogen's effectiveness by assisting in the sensitivity of the estrogen receptors. Young women who are on the BCP for over five years may lose natural estrogen's effectiveness. This is not a true "lack of estrogen" but rather a reduction in its effectiveness. This, in turn, can sometimes be misinterpreted (based on symptoms) as "low estrogen," especially if the woman is in her middle to late thirties. This is one of the reasons that hot flashes can start earlier than would be expected for a woman of this young age. By getting off the BCP (or any synthetic hormone) you will no longer suppress your natural progesterone production and therefore increase your estrogen's effectiveness. Discontinuing the use of the BCP will not only increase your natural progesterone but correct your body's natural system of checks and balances (feedback loops through the hypothalamus and pituitary gland). A restoration of natural hormone production and balance will relieve your PMS symptoms over time.

Heavy bleeding, another familiar symptom of a hormone imbalance, especially seen in young girls, is now becoming more common closer to the menopausal years as well. I increasingly witness this with clients in peri-menopause before the full cessation of their period which occurs in menopause. It is important to address this issue in this chapter because too many women resort to the use of BCP in order to slow or stop excess bleeding.

This heavy bleeding can last as long as ten to twenty days outside of the normal monthly cycle and is caused by extreme "estrogen dominance." Traditionally, if a woman cannot use the BCP, then the medical community will recommend a procedure called an ablation. Generally, this surgery is performed instead of testing the patient's hormones in order to find the root cause of this issue. (An ablation is the removal of the inside of the uterine lining by use of a laser or high-frequency electrical energy, which in turn stops the heavy bleeding).

There have been many success stories for ablations, but there have also been horror stories where there is later more pain involved at menstruation or the procedure does not work at all. What an ablation *does not* do is balance the hormones, which is the root cause for this condition. If you are estrogen dominant and progesterone deficient, your uterine lining can build up too much, leading to the excessive bleeding. Temporary use of the BCP (or an ablation) might put a stop to this but it is not highly recommended since the true hormonal imbalance is not resolved, just masked. Of course, true hormonal balance is the best solution.

Hopefully, it is now clear that hormones can be balanced naturally and the monthly cycle can move along smoothly without the annoying symptoms of PMS (mood swings, cramps, heavy bleeding, etc.). I feel that women should not have to dread their monthly menstrual periods. The BCP is a way to accomplish this but only for a matter of time because it is only masking your symptoms. Underlying imbalances are caused with its use and these subclinical issues will allow your symptoms to eventually resume while increasing other risks. Finding natural balance between estrogen and progesterone, coupled with addressing adrenal fatigue/exhaustion, will be what allows you to become symptom-free for life. You will feel significantly better than simply choosing to mask your symptoms through the use of the BCP. Your body will become healthier and your bothersome monthly symptoms will fade away. Overall, and in due time, the quality of your life will improve without the added risks associated with the synthetic hormones in the BCP. Please refer to Chapter 8 for more specific information on how to naturally balance your hormones to ease PMS symptoms *your very next cycle!*

CHAPTER 6

The Hormone Shift & Mood

The Use of Psychotropic Drugs to Treat Symptoms . . .

What is the connection between the hormone shift and mood? Why are women prescribed psychotropic drugs for their mood issues? Why are there no pre-testing procedures or specific protocols for prescribing psychotropic drugs?
Can depression/anxiety be linked to hormonal shift s that occur monthly, post-partum or around menopause?
Solution: Balance hormones to naturally aid in mood stabilization
Specifics on a natural hormone balancing solution (refer to Chapter 8)

O ver the past decade, the number of people being treated with strong psychotropic drugs for depression/anxiety has significantly increased. In order to classify depression/anxiety as a real disease-state, these conditions are now deemed as a simple imbalance of brain chemicals with no apparent origin—at least the pharmaceutical companies do not appear to be in a rush to pinpoint one. This fact is causing many women, whom are concerned with their health and well-being, to ask the question, "Are psychotropic drugs such as Prozac, Paxil, and Zoloft the most effective treatment for mood swings and feelings of depression/anxiety?"

My twenty-five years of experience in the health field points me to answer a resounding, "No!" Psychotropic drugs, if used without supporting the endocrine (hormonal) system or addressing other emotional and lifestyle factors, will rarely cause mood stabilization to the point a woman feels fully "cured" of her condition. All cases of depression/anxiety that have come through my health center have been connected to adrenal fatigue/exhaustion and the resulting sex hormone imbalance of "estrogen dominance" which is a progesterone deficiency (discussed in Chapter 1). Even if genetics plays a role in this condition, there is also a cause-and- effect origin point. By pinpointing the origin, the condition becomes much more understandable. This allows for a logical treatment and often the permanent cessation of symptoms. In this chapter, I will be discussing depression/anxiety more from the perspective of women's health.

It is an obvious problem that psychotropic drugs are being doled out like candy for depression and anxiety—and this problem is two-fold. 1) These drugs are being prescribed to women without the specific protocols or pre-testing that other drugs require. 2) These drugs are prescribed without a complete explanation of how they work on certain neuro- chemicals (brain chemicals), which happens because this topic is still vastly misunderstood. It just makes sense that there should at least be a simple exploration of common hormonal imbalances prior to a woman being prescribed these strong psychotropic drugs. These imbalances are so easily tied to the irritability of PMS, post-partum depression, and menopausal mood swings. After addressing this hormonal imbalance, simple healthy lifestyle changes coupled with therapy, can bring an even faster and deeper resolution; therefore, strong drugs can oftentimes be avoided.

To start, let us take a look at the seemingly complex issue of depression/ anxiety by discussing both the physical and emotional components in order to determine the origin of this condition. It is impossible to separate the physical from the emotional and act as if this condition is a totally physical state of disease—just like it is impossible to separate the mind from the brain—and yet pharmaceutical companies are referring to depression/ anxiety in this way. By taking a holistic approach, we can work with the body and mind together so that you may fully heal.

Two Important Questions to Ask Yourself:

1. Do you think this feeling you are experiencing is a long-term case of depression/anxiety; where nothing excites you, you have no motivation or desire to do anything, you want to stay sequestered and sleep all the time, or you have experienced a

nervous breakdown or collapse? This scenario is closer to a true mental imbalance and some would argue that psychotropic drugs are warranted.

2. Do you think this feeling you are experiencing is simply a mood shift related to an emotionally stressful life situation, which along with other stressors could have caused adrenal fatigue/exhaustion and a sex hormonal imbalance? This could happen monthly at menstruation, possibly after pregnancy, or have its definable onset after the age of 35-40 when the peri-menopausal or menopausal years begin.

Only you can answer these questions. However, they can serve as a starting point to make you really think about your specific case. Your answer can serve as a basis for treatment options. Unfortunately, there are no readily available and conclusive tests for measuring neuro-chemicals. It is not like measuring your cholesterol or blood sugar. Another problem is that there is no standardization of how to prescribe psychotropic drugs and no baseline testing. When these feelings of depression/anxiety become chronic, women usually seek help from an outside source (like a doctor) and the treatment option is typically a drug prescription—rarely is counseling or hormonal testing recommended.

For the purpose of this chapter, we will refer to "clinical" depression/anxiety as that which has been a chronic case lasting for months or years. An acute case of depression/anxiety is more short-term in nature. This will serve as a basis for our discussion on how a temporary life stressor or situation (divorce, job loss, etc.) Can turn an acute case of depression/anxiety into a chronic or "clinical" case. You will see, however, as the chapter unfolds, that hormone imbalances are involved in both cases.

Hormones Do Affect Our Mood

In my observation of thousands of women, I have seen the majority of cases of chronic depression/anxiety as hormonal in nature. Once estrogen and progesterone are balanced and the adrenal gland is supported, mood issues such as depression/anxiety resolve quite naturally and women can easily wean off of their psychotropic medication—under their doctor's supervision, of course. As explained in previous chapters, hormonal issues worsen with chronic stress. Over time, this will cause irritability and moodiness, and for a certain predisposed group, this can evolve into a "clinical" or chronic case of depression/anxiety. From my experience and in my comparisons of lab tests, I have noticed that if a woman has chronic depression/anxiety, she will also have a hormonal imbalance. My clients fill out a simple hormone questionnaire (like the one in Chapter 1) as their first step toward relief of typical symptoms of PMS or menopause. When they fill out this questionnaire, it is common for them to circle depression and/or anxiety or mood swings as a symptom of concern. However, when women come to me specifically for help with depression/anxiety or mood swings, they always have other symptoms circled that indicate a hormonal imbalance as well. This can be seen without expensive saliva or blood lab testing but just through the commonality of symptoms. There is an undeniable connection here that cannot be ignored by the medical community or anyone looking to treat these conditions. The connection between hormones and depression/anxiety is as such:

- Women often feel "blue," depressed/anxious, or more irritable three to seven days before their period. This is where there tends to be the greatest imbalance of estrogen to progesterone when stress levels are high (example of an acute case of depression/ anxiety).

- Many women go into a period of post-partum depression after having a baby when their hormones are then shift ing back after pregnancy (an example of an acute case of depression/anxiety that can turn chronic).

- Women often experience depression/anxiety for years before the full cessation of their period/ovulation and during menopause (an example of a chronic case of depression/anxiety).

Is this all a coincidence or are these hormonal imbalances or "shift s" connected to or even the key trigger to feelings of depression/ anxiety? We tend to blame these imbalances for our occasional "bitchy" attitude during our PMS week and some lawyers have even made cases that severe PMS, called PMDD (premenstrual dysphoric disorder), can serve as a legitimate basis for certain crimes of passion. So why on earth would we not link these vast hormonal swings and "shift s" to cases of depression/anxiety?

Medicating Moods

Even though it may seem like depression and anxiety are on two opposite ends of the continuum—one is overly excitatory (anxiety) and the other is more of a paralyzed state (depression)—they are actually closely related, and it is common for people to bounce back and forth between the two states of mind. To clarify, anxiety can be looked at as the initial "panic" reaction to a stressful situation, while depression is a "hopelessness" that can set in after the person feels like they cannot control it or overcome it. It is only after a long period of anxiety, brought on by chronic stress, when a true "clinical" or chronic depression occurs (more on this later in the chapter).

Approximately thirty percent of the women I work with are on psychotropic drugs when they first come to see me. Most of these women confess that they do not want to be on these medications, but unfortunately they do not know what else to do for their feelings of depression/anxiety. When I ask, "How is the medication working for you?" almost all of them say something like, "It's okay, I still have my good days and bad days" or "I feel less stressed but less emotional about everything and don't really like the feeling." In other words, if a drug anesthetizes you to pain, it will also have the same effect on pleasure. For most people, this is really not a long-term solution. It makes me wonder if they are any better off on these drugs since it is common to have good and bad days when not on drugs—it is called simply living life. This is something to really think about because there are strong placebo effects associated with many drugs, but this seems especially true in the arena of psychotropic drugs.

A new study published in JAMA (see references) concluded that for the cases of PTSD (post traumatic stress disorder), treatment with Selective Serotonin Reuptake Inhibitor (SSRI) medications proved no better than a placebo. In agreement with this, Irving Kirsch Ph.D., author *The Emperors New Drugs: Exploding the Antidepressant Myth,* (2009) delves further into how many of these drugs received FDA approval on hairline advantages over placebos for symptoms of depression. He goes on to expose the way psychotropic drug manufacturers can hide studies and "water down" negative drug results. Kirsch explains that only a mere two clinical trials are needed to show a psychotropic drug has marginal improvement over a placebo in order to get a new drug on the market (even though many studies may show the drug to be no better than a placebo). Kirsch even accounts for the few studies where a psychotropic drug slightly beat a placebo in effectiveness solely due to participants "breaking blind." This term denotes that participants figured out they were on the real drug (not placebo) because they began to experience the side effects that only the real drug would induce. This common occurrence is influential and has been proven in studies to affect how a participant reports overall "improvement" in their depression/anxiety. There have been several other books by noted psychiatrists on the topic of the misuse and the misunderstanding of psychotropic drugs—they even reveal how the risks far outweigh the benefits. These are bold statements, but may even be understatements. No one really knows what the long-term results are when you push your neuro- chemicals in one direction or another through this type of drug therapy. Dr. Robert Stein, PhD., specializing in neurobehavioral psychology and founder of the Center for Neurobehavioral Health said in an interview with me, "People need to understand that when you take a foreign chemical (a drug) the body, seeking homeostasis, or allostasis, will adjust to that medicine and any beneficial effects may disappear with time, along with long-term changes in synaptic transmission, number of receptors, and receptor sensitivity. Psychotropic medication is too often used in a shotgun approach for mood issues such as depression and anxiety."

This new onslaught of books, recent studies and professional opinions should cause us to think twice before popping these strong drugs. It is yet another reason to consider checking hormone levels first. You will see as you read on how I will directly tie any possible neuro-chemical imbalance directly to an underlying hormone imbalance. This does not mean that I am taking a strong stance against all psychotropic drugs at all times. The main focus of this chapter is that hormonal balance is essential for long-term mood stabilization enhanced by some healthy lifestyle changes. We know depression/ anxiety are real issues, but we need to question the unregulated way that these conditions are being addressed through the use of strong psychotropic drugs—especially when the real cause-and-effect is not actively sought out. These chronic, and often debilitating mood issues, usually will not naturally improve with time unless hormones are balanced and/or a stressful life situation changes. There are also other lifestyle and emotional factors that precede these conditions or are strongly influenced by them, which we will discuss later in the chapter. You will see a vast improvement in the way that you act and the way that you make decisions when you are no longer depressed or anxious. From this point, most life situations can be better dealt with and worked through—and they will not seem as overwhelming!

Let us dive a little deeper into how neuro-chemical and hormonal imbalances that affect our mood tend to start in the first place. This will help you understand your current bout with depression/anxiety and assure you that these symptoms do not have to continually occur in life as you encounter stress. Then, I will provide some guidance on how to handle both physical and hormonal issues along with the mental and emotional issues.

Stress and Neuro-chemicals

Chronic stress can affect the body's hormonal balance, as well as the brain's delicate neuro-chemical balance. In the pages to come it will unfold how the same "fight or flight" reaction produced in us by stress drains the "calming" (inhibitory) hormones and neuro-chemicals leaving an improper ratio of "stimulating" (excitatory) hormones and neuro -chemicals. In short, this stress reaction we experience daily wears on our adrenal gland leading to adrenal fatigue and then later adrenal exhaustion. In other words, the balance of the body has "shift ed" and this leaves us in an imbalanced state that does not feel good! Neuro-chemicals mirror hormones; and therefore, it would not be likely for you to experience a long-term neuro-chemical imbalance without an underlying hormone imbalance. From all I have seen, it does take a longer time for neuro-chemicals to truly shift into a state of imbalance. This is why a hormonal imbalance should be addressed before considering strong psychotropic drugs.

Let us now explore further how neuro-chemicals can shift and lead to serious mood symptoms. As stated above, neuro-chemicals and hormones seem to parallel each other in the body. To oversimplify things, think of neuro-chemicals as being in your brain and hormones being in your body (they actually both work in both areas). Remember from Chapter 1—that when you are under daily stress, your elevated demand for the stress hormone, cortisol, will end up draining your progesterone levels. This will then leave you with an estrogen and progesterone imbalance called "estrogen dominance," which causes all PMS and menopausal symptoms. This phenomenon is paralleled in the brain chemistry with two major neuro-chemicals as well.

Dopamine is a neuro -chemical known to keep us happy, motivated, and energetic; but also helps us to think clearly and feel "on top of the world." Serotonin, on the other hand, is the neuro-chemical governing sleep and appetite, but it is often mistakably touted as the "happy" neuro -chemical because it plays a strong role in our impulse control. It can be associated with happiness because your serotonin is what prevents you from making rash or hasty decisions in regard to that person who just cut you off on the freeway. Let me put it this way . . . serotonin can help keep you out of jail!

Dopamine and serotonin are two of the main neuro-chemicals I will address. They are balanced on sort of a "see-saw." If one goes up, over time, the other tends to go down. This is because the amino acids from which they are made (tryptophan and tyrosine) are known to compete with each other in their crossing of the blood brain barrier. If one is in, the other is out. Over a period of time, stress can create an imbalance of dopamine to serotonin, causing a depressed state. This is directly due to dopamine being lowered, which allows serotonin to be chronically elevated. Neuro -chemicals react to chronic stress and can become imbalanced just as sex hormones react to stress and become imbalanced.

When under stress, the body not only needs to produce the hormone, cortisol, but also needs to produce the neuro-chemicals, adrenaline and norepinephrine. Adrenaline and norepinephrine are "fight-or-flight" chemicals that are literally made out of our dopamine reserves. Constant demand for adrenaline and norepinephrine, due to long-term stress, can eventually cause a drop in dopamine levels. Eventually, you are left with chronically low dopamine (not so happy) and elevated serotonin, resulting in more of a "clinical" depression (see Figure 6 -1). This typically does not happen overnight or with a specific stressful situation that crops up (job loss, divorce, etc.) but would take months or years of stress. Adrenal fatigue is the first condition you will experience combined with a sex hormone imbalance. Later, if stress continues with the sex hormone imbalance left unchecked, adrenal exhaustion can set in. This stage is more likely connected to actual "clinical" depression where there is a true shift in neuro-chemicals. Also, note that adrenal exhaustion would be more likely connected to "second level" hormone depletion (see Chapter 1).

Figure 6-1 Imbalances in Neuro-chemicals

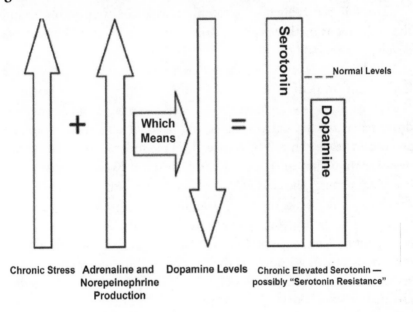

Chronic Stress   Adrenaline and   Dopamine Levels   Chronic Elevated Serotonin —
Norepeinephrine   possibly "Serotonin Resistance"
Production

Bent Formby Ph.D., coauthor of the book Lights Out, was kind enough to provide me with further clarification on serotonin since so many people hear that lowered serotonin levels in the brain are linked to depression, rather than the chronically elevated levels as stated here. This misunderstanding is because most drugs, promoted to supposedly aid in depression (SSRI drugs; example Prozac), actually increase available levels of serotonin. In an interview, Dr. Formby was able to clarify the amazing phenomena of how our dopamine levels drop over time in reaction to elevated stress levels, which automatically leads to our serotonin levels elevating. Initially, this increased serotonin will be read by the body as panic (your initial anxiety) and then when panic never lets up, a depressed state of hopelessness usually follows. His brilliant theory is based on years of research and observation, as well as a multitude of National Institutes of Health (NIH) studies. This theory of chronically high serotonin makes logical sense. It incorporates the idea that depression/anxiety occurs because serotonin is no longer able to work as efficiently in the brain due to a "resistance" that occurs from chronically elevated levels. This is similar to how insulin becomes less effective when it is chronically high, eventually leading to the possibility of diabetes.

To aid in clarifying how "serotonin resistance" can possibly occur in the brain, let us further explore the example of how "insulin resistance" develops in the body.

We know that eating sugars or starches raise our blood sugar, which leads to an immediate release of insulin in order to lower our blood sugar (insulin assists the movement of sugar into our cells). Most people do not realize that caffeine, nicotine, alcohol and stress also cause an insulin release in the bloodstream. This means that even stressful negative thoughts can trigger a rise in insulin! Eventually, when this keeps happening, the cells get "tired" of seeing insulin hanging out all the time—kind of like the pesky neighbor hanging outside your door all the time. Eventually, you are not so thrilled for the company and do not even want to open the door. When the cells no longer "open the door" to take in sugar, this is known as the start of "insulin resistance." "Insulin resistance" is when insulin does not work as efficiently, which results in elevated blood sugar levels for a longer period of time. Unfortunately, when the body becomes insulin resistant, the cells do not readily get the sugar (energy) they need. This situation causes low energy and increases sugar cravings—eventually leading to the potential for the development of full-blown diabetes.

A similar situation can occur with our neuro-chemical, serotonin. If serotonin levels stay high for too long, a "serotonin resistance" can take place and our serotonin cannot get into the brain cells in order to calm us during our stressful times. The root cause of this is the lowered dopamine levels that occur when stress depletes our "happy" neuro-chemical, dopamine. The "see-saw" effect takes over when dopamine levels go down, allowing serotonin levels to build up. This building up of serotonin (outside the cell) over time causes resistance; therefore, it cannot efficiently get into the brain cells to have its intended "calming" effect on us (see Figure 6-2).

Figure 6-2

Stress and the Development of Chronic Depression/Anxiety

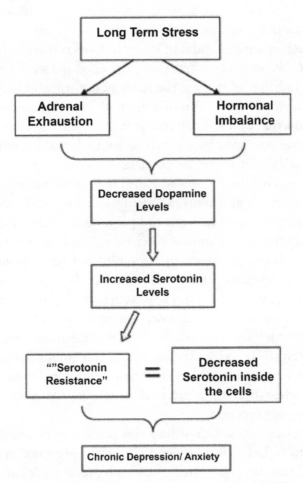

This is where the restlessness, irritability and anxiety set in; and then over a long period of time, depression takes over. Because we are unaware of how sugars and starches can affect our mood, we keep grabbing for the pretzels or candy hoping to get the calm feeling that we need. However, we cannot really pacify our panic at this point by simply eating sugars and starches. It is a temporary "fix" at best.

Hopefully, this logical explanation removes some of the mystery, and can help you to feel empowered as you face your situation of chronic depression/anxiety.

Dr. Formby's book, *Lights Out*, outlines how our hormones can get "out of whack" from our stressful modern society. Over time, this can result in mood issues, as well as many chronic health issues. He explains that this takes place from lack of sleep, but also from the over-consumption of starches and simple sugars. Does this sound like a lot of Americans? We are overworked, tired, depressed and we definitely have hormonal imbalances that are the result of our stressful lifestyles. Dr. Formby's advice in this book is to "sleep it off" because excess serotonin can be converted by the body into melatonin during sleep. This can help to bring serotonin back down to levels that allow our "happy" neuro-chemical, dopamine, to rise. I agree that we need to put down the chips, turn off the TV and go to bed to improve our overall mood. Adequate sleep will also allow the adrenal gland to repair and this will have a positive effect on estrogen and progesterone balance as well!

One surefire way to know if you have reached the point of clinical depression (chronic elevation in serotonin) is when you notice that nothing seems to excite you. You may also lack the motivation or desire to do anything, you want to stay sequestered or sleep all the time, or (in an extreme case), you have had a nervous breakdown or collapse. (This is the body "making" you take some downtime from your "hamster wheel" stressful lifestyle). By this point, you would have definitely been under long-term stress and will have a hormonal imbalance (and exhausted adrenal gland), which both need to be addressed in order to start the healing process.

Now, let us take a look at how this imbalance of hormones, and the subsequent imbalance of neuro-chemicals, plays out in a real life situation. Let us say you started a new high pressure sales job, working for a highly demanding boss. Initially, you would be stressed all of the time from having to reach your sales numbers. Your boss may pop in your office on a daily basis in order to check on your progress. This, in turn, makes you feel on edge. As a matter of fact, you might feel on edge all day as you never know when he may stop by to check on you. You work long hours, barely having time to eat and even when you are off work, you cannot seem to stop thinking about how you will generate more sales. Sometimes at night, you cannot sleep and you spend your time wondering if you will fall below your expected numbers and maybe even be fired. This is a period of extreme mental/ emotional stress and your body is pumping out adrenaline and norepinephrine to keep up with the pace of your stressful lifestyle. This overproduction of adrenaline and norepinephrine begins to drain your dopamine levels, which you eventually start to notice because you certainly do not feel "happy" anymore, even when you are not at work. Of course, while this is happening, cortisol was also being produced; taxing your adrenal gland and draining your progesterone levels, causing a sex hormone imbalance. In this state, all of the pesky PMS or menopausal (depending on your age) symptoms are present and they tend to exacerbate your mental stress from your new job. You have obvious "physical stress" (from lack of sleep, eating too many carbohydrates, from sitting too long, etc.) in addition to all of your mental stress from work. You now start to feel the deeper emotional stress provoking thoughts like, "Why am I doing this? Did I make a mistake with this job? Is this really my passion in life?" This is the initial phase of anxiety that occurs before a true clinical depression sets in. Through this example, I am trying to show you that in a true case of clinical depression (imbalance of neuro-chemicals), a period of long-term stress/anxiety composed of many mental, physical and emotional factors would have to precede it. This has been my observation from working with women and it makes sense especially with knowing how the body functions under stress.

To reiterate, in this example, poor nutrition (too much sugar and starch), lack of sleep, increased physical pain, as well as mental/ emotional stress; causes burnout, which you may have experienced. From this, you seem to move like a "zombie" through the next several weeks and seem to not care anymore. You want to sleep in and have to struggle to get out of bed in the morning. There is no joy in anything you do and you may even consider irrational or radical things (quit your job, move away, check yourself in somewhere, or commit suicide). This would be an example of clinical depression where the sex hormones are imbalanced (low progesterone) and the adrenal gland exhausted, coupled with the neuro- chemicals having shift ed to a point of lowered dopamine and elevated serotonin. Both of these neuro-chemicals are important and need to be in balance for us to feel our best, just like balancing estrogen to progesterone levels as described throughout this book.

As you can see, drained dopamine levels and drained progesterone levels mirror each other in this simplified example. This shows that you would have to have imbalanced hormones if neuro-chemicals were truly out of balance. It would only make sense that after exciting your nervous system through a stressful re-occurring life situation, it will become trained to be in the "fight-or-flight" mode, which works off of your sympathetic nervous system. This part of the nervous system was only meant to be triggered when you are ready for real danger. When we are relaxing, or not perceiving danger, our bodies function in the parasympathetic nervous system, which allows us to digest our food and rebuild our body tissue. In this state, the immune system functions optimally. Both the sympathetic and the parasympathetic systems are an important part of the autonomic nervous system that runs our bodies. You see, the body totally "shift s" gears and its priorities when it thinks it is in danger—raiding our precious reserves of enzymes, hormones and neuro-chemicals. When this occurs it can lead to disease, depression/anxiety, and rapid aging. Chronic fatigue, fibromyalgia, certain cancers, and autoimmune diseases are often precipitated by months or even years of chronic stress.

A Theory on the "Origin" of Depression/Anxiety

By this point, you probably understand the importance of balancing your sex hormones as a foundation for feeling better as you deal with the emotional issues related to your depression/anxiety. This process involves working on balancing your estrogen and progesterone while dealing with the stress and adrenal fatigue/exhaustion that started the whole process. There are quick and easy solutions to these imbalances, which are mentioned in Chapter 8. However, I would like to go a bit deeper for those of you who truly want more answers about why you may be suffering from chronic depression/anxiety, while others, who have the same hormonal imbalance, are not.

The brain can either drive (push) the mind into an imbalanced state or the mind can drive (push) the brain into an imbalanced state—where the imbalance of neuro-chemicals and hormones will lead to feelings of depression/anxiety. The brain is like our hardware and it works with the "chemistry" of the body being affected by sleep, nutrition and hormones. The mind is a bit harder to get our hands around but it acts more like the software or program that runs our brain's computer. It is the intangible system that works on energy and relates more to the "physics" of the body. The two following scenarios both point to the fact that the issue of depression/anxiety is not simply a physical neuro-chemical imbalance alone:

Two Scenarios to Consider:

Scenario I, *"The Brain Driving the Mind "* into an imbalanced state: Physical factors, such as an inherited hormonal imbalance or disadvantage, causes an overly sensitive "fight-or-flight" response that negatively affects your thought patterns; a physical origin then affecting your mental/ emotional well-being.

Scenario II, *"The Mind Driving the Brain"* into an imbalanced state: Mental factors, such as thoughts and your attitude (related to a life situation) causes stress and drains the body's hormones and neuro-chemicals over time; a mental/emotional origin then affecting your physical well-being.

Dawn M. Cutillo

Figure 6-2

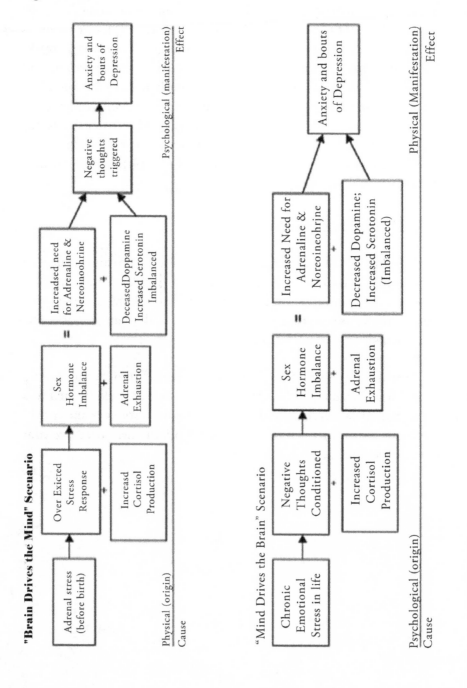

Both imbalanced scenarios originate from chronic stress—either physical (hormones) or mental/emotional (thoughts/attitude). These scenarios are depicted in Figure 6-3. Even the allopathic medical community verifies that stress affects our health, and in America, most stress has its origin in mental thoughts and emotions. At some point, this stress will need to be dealt with in order to achieve true healing at the core level. If you can determine the source of the stress, it will aid you in pinpointing the origin of your depression/anxiety. The next two sections should help you understand what is at play in your particular case so that you can better understand your situation.

Scenario I—The "Brain Driving the Mind" into a State of Imbalance

A chemical imbalance in the brain can start at birth. The brain works with the chemistry of the body; and therefore, it can be susceptible to imbalances caused by stress. Most often, the imbalance at birth comes from a mother's stress (physical or emotional) during pregnancy. This can also occur due to toxins (such as heavy metals) that enter the fetus from the mother's body or toxins that enter into the baby via the breast milk. Any kind of stress that the mother may deal with during her pregnancy—either temporarily excessive or chronic— will affect the brain chemistry of the developing fetus and can shift it to an imbalance of a higher proportion of excitatory neuro-chemicals and a lower proportion of sedating/calming neuro-chemicals. This is usually because the mother's body utilizes and drains the fetus' adrenal hormones. The resulting effect is the imbalance of hormones and neuro-chemicals in the developing child. When a person comes from this inherited disadvantage, it can seem impossible to overcome their chronic depression/anxiety. This should not be classified as a true genetic disorder as it stems from a very specific cause-and-effect scenario, which offers hope of resolution.

In this situation, adrenal fatigue/exhaustion results in the brain's imbalance of neuro -chemicals and will drive the mind into negative or unhealthy thought patterns that are self-generated. If you have more of an inherited imbalance in brain chemistry (from birth or as long as you can remember) this will often cause you to be extremely sensitive in your thought patterns in relation to any emotional stressors. This can then cause you to lament easily over relatively small issues, which creates a vicious cycle. These stressful thoughts conjured in the mind will drive the brain's neuro-chemicals into more of an imbalance. Again, the "fight-or-flight" response is triggered easily and more often than it should be in a day's time. We have this "fight-or-flight" response to protect us from the chance of real danger of death or injury, which in our modern society, we do not run into on a daily basis. However, in this situation, for a person who has weakened brain chemistry, their mind will cause them to perceive a thought as if it was real stress, and the "fight-or-flight" response kicks in.

If this is your situation, you could appear to be highly emotional, moody, or seem to "take things to heart easily," but there is a physiological origin and reason for these feelings. This is not your innate personality but a highly sensitive and often addictive stress response to which your body has grown accustomed. This scenario can then be aggravated by lack of sleep, poor nutrition, an unhealthy home environment, difficult childhood, other physical stress factors, and even psychotropic drugs (touched on later in the chapter). Once this overly-sensitive way of feeling or thinking is established, certain thought patterns, or what's termed "neuro-nets" (thought associations between brain cells), begin to form—laying the basis for limiting beliefs in adulthood. A "limiting belief" is simply a thought perspective we have adopted as our own based on things we have observed or were taught by others. It often holds no real truth or validity but tends to alter our behavior and limit our potential. Unfortunately, when ingrained into our thinking, over time it becomes our truth. Both a "limiting belief" and a "neuro-net" can combine and cause a "limiting belief neuro-net." An example would play out like this; every time you step foot into a church you think of your wedding, which makes you think of love, which makes you think of your ex spouse, which makes you remember how he cheated on you, which makes you recall all the pain of the divorce. You have illogically associated a "church" with "pain" from all those connections; but more likely, you associate love with pain by choosing to form specific thought patterns.

If you fit into Scenario I, the negative experiences you have as you go through life will tend to cause more of these "limiting belief neuro-nets" to form. These thought associations will trigger a strong negative reaction within you. Breaking out of this cycle can be almost impossible if you are prone to be pessimistic from weakened brain chemistry. In summary, you have weakened brain chemistry along with an overly-sensitive thought process and many past experiences of negativity to draw from (negative "neuro-nets"). This further validates your chronic thoughts of "pending doom" or "catastrophe." Perhaps you can relate so far. Some people can be so sensitive that they turn any news—which would be totally benign to one person—into a negative scenario, making the situation "permanent and pervasive." An example would be if you miss a call from a friend that you have not heard from in a long time and they do not leave you a voicemail message. Being sensitive, you are sure it is bad news and you play it out into a ridiculous course of catastrophic events, which are all highly unlikely. If this scenario depicts you, much work is now needed for brain chemistry balance so that you can stop easily triggering your "fight-or-flight" (physical) response. Some attention must be spent on breaking through the mind's established thought patterns and "limiting belief neuro-nets" that have formed over the years.

Needless to say, a hormone imbalance is evident and it needs to be addressed for relief. Additionally, disciplined thought, positive reinforcement, relaxation techniques, proper sleep, daily exercise and good nutrition will all aid in breaking this vicious cycle. I will touch more on these lifestyle changes at the end of this chapter. Trying one or two of these suggestions will not be enough if the underlying hormonal imbalance is not addressed.

Scenario I is definitely more rare than Scenario II. Most people with chronic depression tend to fall into Scenario II.

Scenario II—The "Mind Driving the Brain" into a State of Imbalance

If you were born with normal brain chemistry, and were healthy as a child, you can still experience a state of chronic depression/anxiety if the mind constantly triggers negative stressful thoughts based on emotional life situations. This scenario is where the mind (your thoughts) drives the brain's chemistry into a state of imbalance. This is often a result of being in a negative home, relationship, or job situation that causes long-term emotional stress. The new sales job with the high pressure boss, which I previously explained, would be a great example of this pattern. Another more extreme example is PTSD (post traumatic stress disorders)—someone who was at war for weeks or months can experience this. The "mind driving the brain," however, can start at a young age and can result from being raised in a very difficult home environment or perhaps from being beaten, teased or constantly criticized. These situations, or just a general lack of love and support while growing up, can trigger a stress response and cause a negative way of thinking. This means that you can be easily triggered to have negative thoughts when you are faced with life's trying situations. If this is your scenario, you could feel more pessimistic and tend to worry and fret more, but there is an obvious reason; you have been mentally trained to do so based on your past experiences. Also, "limiting belief neuro-nets" are formed from these past experiences and will further aggravate the situation. This negative thinking will put the same drain on your stress and sex hormones and subsequently the neuro-chemicals of the brain. This, in combination with some other factors such as lack of sleep, toxins, and poor nutrition, can cause a neuro-chemical imbalance of chronic low dopamine and slightly elevated serotonin in addition to the pre-existing foundation of adrenal fatigue/exhaustion with a hormonal imbalance of "estrogen dominance."

In another example, to make this point more clear, let us say you grew up in fear of your emotionally abusive, alcoholic father. Protective thoughts, as well as the "fight-or-flight" response become ingrained in your mind so that you tend to react at the very sight of him. Often, this can grow into a reaction that is tipped off at the very mention of your father. The repetition of these excitatory neuro-chemicals and stress hormones being released into the body will place a drain on the sex hormones and needed neuro- chemicals. Soon, anxiety will manifest and long-term depression will eventually result, paralleling the pre-existing adrenal fatigue and sex hormone imbalance.

Which Scenario Do You Relate To?

Determining which scenario you fit into, although not necessary for healing, will aid you tremendously in making sense of all of this.

Since you now know there is an underlying hormonal imbalance, quick and effective progress can be made when you address your adrenal fatigue/exhaustion and your estrogen and progesterone imbalance. This foundation will provide you with clearer thinking; and therefore, a mental edge to deal with your stressful life situation allowing you the motivation to start incorporating some healthy lifestyle changes. Fine-tuning the process by determining the origin, as described above, as well as working on your attitude will help tremendously. If you can indeed determine the cause- and- effect of your depression/anxiety, it will ring true to you and this will help you begin the deepest healing process. Understanding there is always a cause-and- effect to all things in nature is very important. This fact can serve as a relief because it shows that things are not random and chaotic in the Universe and you are not a victim. This does not mean it is your fault or that you should feel guilty for being the cause of your depression/anxiety.

If your depression/anxiety is determined to be a long-term issue of Scenario I—the "brain driving the mind"—this might be an extremely rare case, some would argue, where short-term use of a psychotropic drug may be helpful. Be sure that it is prescribed by a psychiatrist and be sure to work with a good psychologist to break your initial "physical" anxiety or fear cycle that is easily triggered. This is not my initial recommendation by any means; and therefore, it should be taken very seriously as psychotropic drugs are serious. In PTSD and extreme cases of disaster, this treatment option may offer short-term relief. This two-pronged approach will work on the brain and the mind together as both are involved. However, testing your hormone levels or taking the symptom-based questionnaire at the end of Chapter 1 would be a wise first step. If you discover from either of these methods that you have a sex hormone imbalance, I would encourage you to initially try the practical solutions in Chapter 8 because they do not have the side effects that strong psychotropic drugs tend to have. This is a simple protocol I suggest for hormone health—it is logical and will give you enough results to motivate you to make other healthy lifestyle changes (mentioned later in the chapter), which are needed for true long- term healing.

If you determined that your depression/anxiety is more closely related to Scenario II—the "mind-driving the brain"—placing an emphasis on cognitive therapy with a trained psychotherapist and participating in energy work, such as Reiki, will allow you to "let go" of negative emotions. This can prove to be a very powerful combination. By stopping your negative thought patterns, you will naturally lower your mental stress and allow your neuro- chemicals and hormone levels to naturally replenish. The result—you will feel better and be more mentally stable and resilient.

I have even seen some cases where both scenarios have paralleled each other, meaning, weakened brain chemistry was probably present at birth followed by a difficult childhood or other emotional factors that affected the mind. Great improvement is still within reach when a holistic approach to this condition is followed with some discipline. Both scenarios, I and II, or the combination of the two, will respond quickly to natural hormone balancing because in both cases adrenal fatigue/exhaustion has most definitely occurred.

Psychotropic Drugs for Mood Stabilization

There is one last point that must be emphasized on the use of strong psychotropic drugs before we talk more about some healthy practical solutions for mood issues. These drugs, as all drugs do, tend to force the body in a certain direction and sometimes stop symptoms, but often cause more issues with resistance down the road. Based on the new studies and findings that I have already shared, it is questionable if they even work. This is similar to the continued use of synthetic HRT (like estrogen for hot flashes), even though dreaded diseases, such as female cancers, can occur as a result. These "solutions" are simply bandages, and risky ones at that. I have seen cases where psychotropic drugs from a few different sub-categories are layered on top of one another in order to get the desired results. This over prescription by some doctors is ridiculous and potentially dangerous.

Remember that cholesterol, blood pressure, and blood sugar are all meticulously monitored prior to a doctor prescribing medication for their regulation. Currently, even hormone levels are checked before augmenting a woman with bio-identical hormones. However, mind-altering drugs that can totally "mess with" how we think, how we feel, our sex drive and our desire to live—are given out like candy! These drugs are often prescribed based on a few mood complaints that might be mentioned to your family doctor. Certainly, I would be remiss to not recap my opinion on how these drugs are dispensed—this is at the heart of the real controversy. As mentioned before, there are no set protocols for their use, which is obvious to anyone who has a prescription. This is unlike other FDA-approved drugs that are given for thyroid, blood pressure, cholesterol, etc. Use of psychotropic drugs would be more widely accepted if they were explained better to patients, dosed with a temporary plan in mind and used in conjunction with some psychotherapy—and, of course in my opinion, a simple hormone assessment. A protocol should be set to aid general practitioners, who often feel like they are taking a "shot in the dark" by trying different drugs with no real basis. All that doctors have to go off of is what you, as a stressed patient, tell them. This inefficient process can be frustrating for doctors and patients alike.

In my opinion, a general practitioner should not prescribe these strong medications but rather refer the patient to a more experienced psychiatrist who regularly deals with these drugs as a main part of their practice. Psychotropic drugs are usually not life-threatening; however, they certainly can be life-threatening if someone commits suicide while taking them! I almost had this happen to a dear friend of mine who had a hormonal imbalance and a weakened brain chemistry (we later grew to understand), but was put on a commonly prescribed SSRI drug after going through a tough life experience. The reaction to the drug made him very anxious, and then he started to drink excessively to calm himself down (alcohol is a depressant). Weeks later he was put into rehab for drinking, which was never an issue for him in the past, and he almost committed suicide while under the supervision of the medical staff there. He was told years ago that he had a slight issue with bi-polar tendencies (and always dealt with some depression/anxiety) but the doctor who put him on the drug never asked that, even though it clearly states on the precaution information that this drug should not be used with bi-polar patients. You may be wondering why he did not go off the drug when he felt so bad. Well, his doctor and different website blogs said it sometimes takes two weeks to start to feel better and to "stick it out," because you will feel worse, at first, before you feel better. If a mood-altering drug makes you feel "worse first, then better" and there are no scientifically measurable factors in place, it would make sense that you could possibly be tricked into thinking it was finally working when you finally feel better. After two weeks you may be just rising out of your "mental hell" that the drug caused in the first place. This reaction could simply be the result of your body learning to adapt and/or compensate for the drug. Talk about an "emperor's new clothes" scenario! The title of Kirsch's new book could not be more fitting. Maybe this "feeling better" after several weeks on a drug is simply caused by your body finally adapting to it. I guess his friends and family are lucky he went off this drug in rehab in time to preserve his life.

Side note: A theory on how a Selective Serotonin Reuptake Inhibitor (SSRI) drug works proves interesting. This type of drug is designed to add extra serotonin to your system (increasing it or its effects) by preventing its re-uptake (absorption). This is based on the false premise that depression results from low serotonin levels, which incidentally has never been proven in clinical studies. SSRIs can seem effective if you are already high in serotonin (clinical depression), due to the fact that if the body has too much of a chemical or hormone it gives the same result as "not enough," because of a resulting "resistance" to the chemical or hormone. In this situation, you experience a "burnout" to serotonin at the receptor site level which would tend to relieve the symptoms of serotonin "buildup." This idea should now sound familiar. It is the exact same type of effect doctors get with women when putting them on more estrogen to get rid of hot flashes—estrogen is prescribed even when they already have too much estrogen in relation to progesterone (see Chapter 2). The burnout of the estrogen receptor sites will cause a temporary relief of symptoms.

Say you are in the normal range with your brain chemicals, and you take an SSRI drug, maybe due to stress in your life that temporarily has made you upset, or you take it because of mood issues related to a basic sex hormonal imbalance. By taking this drug, serotonin levels can be pushed up to levels equaling that of depression. This is why the precautions often say, "May cause thoughts of suicide in teens or young adults." This makes sense because we all know that children and teens are most often too young to have had enough years of a hormonal imbalance to possibly have caused a true neuro-chemical imbalance. If, however, you are truly to the point that you may be high in serotonin (due to its buildup), you may get the effect of it being lowered due to a "burn-out" to serotonin at the receptor site. This could result in some relief of your symptoms.

This misinformation or lack of education relating to serotonin by drug companies often makes it trickier for doctors when prescribing psychotropic drugs. Therefore, unless a doctor knows for sure that a patient is high in serotonin to begin with (which is not tested for) and that is what is causing the depression, giving an SSRI drug to increase serotonin can cause a further depressed state. Therein lies the danger of these drugs. Suicidal thoughts can be the worst case scenario resulting from a poorly prescribed medicine followed closely by the fact that these drugs are bandaging a deeper hormonal or emotional issue that needs to be addressed.

Keep in mind, using one type of drug to temporarily help you while working on other hormonal or mental issues is one thing. If you feel better on the drug, you know that the doctor nailed it the first time; but remember the recent study showing that it could possibly be related to the placebo effect. If you are not doing well on a drug, check with your doctor to switch to another one, as opposed to adding onto this drug. When you fully understand the few classes of drugs available to you (see Appendix F), more than two types of drugs will either overlap or have a "canceling out" effect. You can only really increase or inhibit neuro-chemicals and there are only basically excitatory and inhibitory neuro-chemicals. I have seen women in my office on four or five different psychotropic drugs at once, with two or more being the same class of drug. In my opinion, it is highly irresponsible to prescribe this way and these women usually feel worse than if they were on no drugs at all! In theory, if the drugs were really working, you should feel increasingly better for each drug that you are on, right? I have helped many women slowly wean off of these drugs through along with their doctor's guidance.

If you still want to consider taking strong psychotropic drugs for depression/anxiety (or are on them now) here are a few helpful hints to determine which direction to go. First and foremost, check your hormone levels to see what this reveals. Then check with your doctor to seek their advice based on what specific issues you are dealing with. This also gives you time to ask for a thorough explanation of what could be causing these issues. From there, you can plan the action you should take. This is basic information that you truly deserve to know. If you do decide to take a prescription drug, be sure to ask your doctor the following questions:

1. Which system is this drug working on? Relaxing/inhibiting excitatory neuro-chemicals (to ease anxiety) or stimulating more excitatory neuro-chemicals (to ease depression). Or, is it a combination of both? What "class" does this drug fall into and what does this class of drug do? (Examples would be SSRI or an SNRI—see classes of drugs in Appendix F).

2. Have you ever used the drug that you are prescribing me for depression/anxiety and for how many years have you had experience with it?

3. What side effects does this drug have based on what the pharmaceutical company says and what side effects have you seen with the use of this drug in your practice?

4. Did the drug representative that explained this drug to you go over any clinical trials and double blind studies on it? Is that information readily available to me, the patient?

5. How long do you estimate I will be on this drug or when can I expect to stop taking it, in your opinion? Does this fit into an overall plan for my health? (For example, the doctor might say, "Please take the drug while you are going through this tough time of losing your job, then you can wean off.")

6. Are there side effects from weaning off this drug?

7. I am taking [fill in the blank—including all drugs, herbs, vitamins, HRT, or the birth control pill]. Will there be any interactions at all with this drug?

8. How do you plan to monitor me on this drug to know if it's working or that the dose is correct for me?

These answers will help you to feel better and assist you in making an informed decision. If your doctor is annoyed with these simple but detailed questions, you might use that as an intuitive tip to find another doctor who goes beyond the superficiality of dolling out drugs without looking at the specific case and the whole person.

Finishing Touches: Working on Mental Factors and Attitudes That Need Shift ing

It may be important for you to determine if your depression is really an imbalance in brain-chemistry or if it is just sadness/ disappointment due to a temporary situation in life that would normally be upsetting. Either of these, or a combination of both, will most often be accompanied by a Shift in your hormones as discussed. An acute depressed state that is now manifesting with physical hormonal and neuro- chemical imbalances will always have an emotional component to it. Examples would be not being fulfilled in your job or in your marriage or simply not liking what you see in the mirror since weight gain or hair loss has occurred. Going deeper, you may find out it could be because you are not living your life authentically, not following your heart, or always doing what others want you to do because it is expected. There is often no real joy in this and sometimes no outlet for your creativity. You can be left with a feeling of emptiness because you do not see your individual fingerprint on this earth, and hence, no way of giving back to the Universe. This is an example of a feeling of being repressed and can over time lead to an inner anger at yourself (or others) that will drive brain chemistry into a depressed state, due to the neuro-chemical imbalance stated above. It has been proven that a poor attitude and negative thoughts lead to negative emotions and this can suppress immune function. This can potentially lead to many diseases and other unhealthy conditions as we age. This phenomenon is now being studied more often and it is becoming more quantifiable.

Recently, it has been discovered that all thoughts provoke emotions that can be associated with certain vibrational frequencies. Dr. Bach, a noted European doctor, studied this and developed homeopathic remedies from flowers that counteract negative thoughts called *Bach Flower Essences*, which have been used in Europe for many years. Noted psychiatrist, Dr. David Hawkins, in the book *Power Vs. Force*, explains the testing for each emotion and how all emotions can be calibrated scientifically to a specific level. Emotions are studied as having a specific effect on the "energy" of our body all the way down to our very atoms and molecules. The higher calibrations, Dr. Hawkins scientifically found, were connected to thoughts and emotions of peace, joy and love. Emotions of anger, fear, guilt and shame were calibrated at very low levels.

It is important to assess your life to determine your level of satisfaction. If you are not satisfied with your life this will create stress that contributes to negative thought patterns leading to negative cycles of emotions. By easing this stress, the result is an eventual rising of your overall vibration or hertz level in the body (explained in Chapter 4). This can be achieved by disciplining the mind while simultaneously dealing with the physical aspects of the brain's chemical imbalance through hormonal therapy. Just as negative thoughts can exacerbate weakened brain chemistry— positive affirmations, meditation, and a good night's sleep have a synergistic effect on supplemental and nutritional support for the brain's neuro-chemical balance. These steps can even be implemented while taking a psychotropic drug. Then, weaning off of this drug becomes not only easy but necessary. I have seen many women become more hormonally balanced while they are on a psychotropic drug, and then these drugs throw them back into an "imbalance" if not weaned off (see Appendix F). This is proven by the anxiety and depression that occurs when a person is on a psychotropic drug and they are not truly in need of it.

Important Steps for Overall Healing

1. Be sure to get your hormones balanced to quickly ease physical symptoms related to your anxiety/depression. (Check the simple hormone analysis at the end of Chapter 1 to see if you are mild, moderate or severe). A symptom-based analysis is often enough, but if you really want to get your hormones tested, opt for saliva testing over blood testing (see resources for a lab). Then consider addressing adrenal exhaustion/fatigue with supplemental support and also supplementing with progesterone.

2. Realize the issue at hand and know that there are many options and pathways to healing. You must explore a few and find what is best for your body. Your intuition, prayer, or meditation on this matter can help in this decision.

3. Decide to consciously change your intentions by the use of daily positive affirmations—even if this means writing them down and reading them out loud. The power of your voice in your own ears is amazing. We always say negative things about ourselves and to others and look where that has taken us, so why not try the positive side of this. Louise Hay has a good book called You Can Heal Your Life, which contains many positive affirmations (see resources).

4. If you failed in your past attempts to beat your chronic depression, negotiate with yourself on why you might still need the depression/ anxiety feelings at this point in your life. Try to pinpoint the reason and learn from it. It sounds crazy, but if the subconscious knows we still need this condition to "define" us, we will remain depressed until we understand this. All diseases (or negatives) have a positive side. I have had women tell me that even though they hate it, their depression "allows" them to get out of doing certain things, gives them more attention from their husbands and serves as the ultimate excuse for why they are not where they should be in life. Know that you are more than this "condition" that seems to define you and that you deserve to be happy.

5. Get enough sleep to balance brain chemistry (eight to nine hours for several weeks, then seven to eight hours when you feel better). Elevated serotonin can be easily brought down by just sleeping. That is why clinically depressed people (literally too much serotonin) will want to sleep all day in an inherent effort to heal. The body will, through sleep, turn excess serotonin to melatonin, which will balance the body and aid you in creating better sleep patterns that continue the healing process.

6. Temporarily stop eating foods that cause a stress response in the body (like gluten in wheat, or casein in milk) as these will

increase your body's need for cortisol production. This will also drain neuro-chemicals by triggering the already too-often-used "fight-or-flight" response. If you determine that you feel better when off of these foods, and then when you add them back into your diet, you feel tired, bloated, have gas or constipation; then you may have a slight food sensitivity to one or both and you may do well to eliminate them from your diet. A digestive enzyme will help as well (more on this in Chapter 8).

7. Keep blood sugar balanced to prevent blood sugar drops throughout the day. Blood sugar imbalances are very stressful to the body and cause us to rev up the "fight-or-flight" response, which can often trigger anxiety and affect overall mood. Below are several ways to keep your blood sugar in check for mood stabilization. I like to say, "How you feel is always connected to your last meal!" Eventually, as you get your blood sugar under control and your hormones become more balanced, you will not be as sensitive to these fluctuations and slight insulin resistance can be reversed.

a. The best way to avoid blood sugar fluctuations is to avoid processed foods or white flour foods like bread, pasta, cakes, muffins, crackers, and so on. This practice will aid in weight management as well. If you want to have these foods, be sure you consume them with protein, fiber or fat as these will slow the uptake of the sugar or carbohydrates in order to keep blood sugar from spiking and then crashing. This process often triggers anxiety, or at least irritability. Limit sweeteners like sugar, honey, maple syrup and agave nectar as these can still spike blood sugar. Artificial sweeteners and herbal stevia, even if no calories are in them, will cause an insulin response or what is called a cephalic (brain) response causing the body to expect sugar even though none is coming. This results in insulin still being released into the bloodstream and leaving you with lower blood sugar and craving more sweets. I found a new fully natural sugar made from fruit that has a low glycemic index and no cephalic response. It is also delicious right out of the jar unlike most artificial sweeteners (see resources).

b. Reduce the amount of chemicals you ingest through processed foods, sodas and alcohol, as well as over-the-counter drugs and prescription medication when you can. (Do not stop or lower prescription medication without getting permission from your doctor.) By lowering these toxins you take stress off of the liver, which will always aid in overall blood sugar balance.

c. Increase protein throughout the day to aid in balancing out blood sugar from the carbohydrates consumed. Eat a small source of protein every three hours until you get this issue under control. Or, if you do want to eat something with sugar in it, consume it with some protein to avoid a blood sugar spike, which is followed by a fall that may irritate your mood. An example would be a hardboiled egg, some nuts or seeds, or even a protein bar or shake.

d. Increase good fats that heal the body. Another way to keep blood sugar steady is with good fats, like flax and fish oil, as these are excellent for brain chemistry. Consider an overall Omega oil blend, made from all three essential fatty acids like Omega 3, 6 and 9 for better balance. Also, the medium chain triglycerides in coconut oils are healthy, aid in weight loss and will burn slowly; keeping blood sugar balanced.

e. Stop caffeine, if at all possible (or only drink one cup of tea/coffee in the morning), as this will also trigger a stress response in the body with cortisol going up, then the resulting blood sugar rise and fall (due to insulin being released) can often trigger anxiety. Consider herbal teas or even green tea (low caffeine, high in antioxidants) or white or red rooibos tea (no caffeine). I have found a coffee that I recommend to my clients that has patented "buffered" caffeine. It was developed by a doctor who performs glycemic index testing for the government. This will not only allow for smoother blood sugar transitions and more even moods, but it also promotes fat-burning because no excess sugar is released into the blood stream unlike during the normal cortisol response that regular coffee provokes (see resources).

8. Exercise—Get physical. Get out of your head and focus more on the physical aspects of yourself, not just the mental realm of negative thoughts. Less intense exercise is preferred here; focus on exercises like calisthenics, Pilates, yoga and weight training. These exercises are preferred for an anxious/depressed person. Too much high intensity aerobic exercise can cause a "fight-or-flight" cortisol response, triggering anxiety. Think of prehistoric times— they "ran" when being chased, not for exercise. Running also tends to be hard on your joints as you age. Dancing (which is fun and joyful) will not evoke the same stress response, nor will walking, and therefore these types of exercises are healthier for the adrenal gland.

9. Have daily quiet time for prayer, meditation or contemplation, preferably mid to late afternoon after work, or right before bed if no other time will work. Mid-day is best because it can ease stress for the rest of the day. Try a relaxation CD that uses brainwave synchronization music to relax brainwave patterns from a stressed state to a relaxed state (more on this in Chapter 8). This form of "sound therapy" takes only 20-30 minutes and allows you to feel as if you got two hours of sleep (see resources).

10. Stay busy and have a fun hobby or creative outlet you can do daily. Boredom can breed negative thoughts and build up stress hormones like cortisol, causing physical aches and pains. This certainly is not helpful in motivating you to move more!

Point to remember: *A healthy lifestyle will lead to a healthy mind and brain chemistry!*

In conclusion, I would like to say there is hope even for seemingly severe depression/anxiety, and I trust you feel the same way after reading this chapter. The body naturally strives for balance, or homeostasis. This applies to hormones and the delicate balance of brain chemicals that affect our mood. Our attempt to live outside the laws of health and balance in our fast-paced society can eventually lead to symptoms of depression/anxiety and disease. The stress of our lifestyle, here in America, and the busy schedule it demands from us, are the main causes of a shift in hormones. This then causes an imbalance of the neuro-chemicals dopamine and serotonin leading to the more rare cases of true clinical depression/anxiety.

As you become healthier by practicing the steps listed above, your brain chemistry will shift in the right direction. Simple steps such as more sleep, twenty minutes of daily meditation, and proper nutrition can make a lasting impact. Determining the root cause of how your chronic depression/anxiety started will also aid you in healing and preventing it from reoccurring. Balancing your hormones and lowering stress, to ensure this balance holds, is one of the best places to start and I offer detailed solutions in Chapter 8.

We all have times of unhappiness or temporarily being in a bad mood, but if our hormones are balanced, we are much more resilient to the ramifications of our daily "crazy" schedules or the larger life trials that can get us down. Please look at the approach to your mental health as multifaceted and attempt some of the suggestions given here. Realize that although you may still choose to temporarily use a psychotropic drug, this will often not be a true healing path because the body is still out of balance hormonally from stress and poor lifestyle choices. And of course, an attitude check is important because how we look at our situation is always part of determining the outcome. After digesting this information, I know you will be more likely to look at your situation with hope and not despair, then you can reap the added benefits that a positive attitude has on healing.

CHAPTER 7

The Hormone Shift & Aging

The Use of HGH to Slow the Aging Process . . .

What happens in the body hormonally as we age?
Why do we seem like we are aging faster in our modern world?
Is the use of "anti-aging" hormones safe and/or effective?
Solution: Supplement with an "anti-aging" hormone (HGH) and make lifestyle changes to slow aging naturally
Specifics on using HGH for natural hormone balancing (refer to Chapter 8)

As we age in a society that values youth, many people find themselves wondering, "Is it unsafe or unnatural to try to slow the aging process? Is it just plain vain? Is replenishing an 'anti-aging' hormone (like HGH) tampering with Mother Nature?"

From a purely world-view standpoint, the answer would be, "No." It is becoming more evident that we are aging prematurely as our main youth hormone "shift s" due to our fast-paced, high-stress lifestyle in America. This is also exacerbated by the over-consumption of sugar and caffeine, and by the contamination of our food with chemicals and toxins. These factors cause our human growth hormone (HGH) levels to drain abnormally early, speeding up the aging process and slowing cell replication. The good news is that HGH can be safely and cost-effectively replaced so that the aging process is slowed and even reversed to an extent. This result can simply be accomplished with the synergistic combination of HGH and some basic lifestyle changes. This provides support to the body's endocrine system. Human growth hormone (HGH), as described in Chapter 1, is produced by somatotropic cells in the anterior pituitary gland located deep within the brain. It is the most abundant hormone produced by this gland—over forty percent of the cells in the pituitary gland are somatotropic cells.

Sometimes called the "master hormone," the role of HGH is to:

1. **Affect nearly every cell in the body as a child grows;** When we are young our pituitary gland excretes HGH causing us to grow and mature. For example, it aids in the completion of our long bone between the ages of twenty and twenty-five.

2. **Slow the aging process in an adult's cells by helping them regenerate, repair, and replicate themselves;** If HGH is working properly, new cells form as old cells die; therefore, healthy cells are constantly replacing unhealthy cells!

Theory of Aging and Loss of HGH in the Body

As we age, our pituitary gland loses its "motivation" and instead of establishing a balanced level, HGH begins to steadily decrease. At the age of sixty, its effectiveness is only twenty percent of what it was in our twenties. The steady decline is called "somatopause" (like menopause) and decreases at a rate of twenty percent per decade.

The question is, "Why does this happen?" We do not have a death gene. Our cells are proven to easily live up to one hundred and twenty years, and in other countries, some people live to be over one hundred years old. It would make sense that the more we know about why this hormone declines rapidly, the better chance there is to prevent premature aging.

The hypothalamus gland is directly affected by the emotional stress of the body. It normally tells the pituitary gland to produce HGH via a negative feedback system, meaning when HGH gets low in the blood, the hypothalamus will tell the pituitary gland to produce more of it. We know that the hypothalamus can be "thrown off" if the body is being chronically overstressed. This can cause the inability to lose weight and to normally gain weight. The European physician,

Dr. Simeons, who is discussed in Chapter 3, brought this information to light in the 1930's through his research on the hypothalamus. The mental and/or emotional stress we encounter daily, coupled with our consumption of an overabundance of sugar and toxins, further compounds this problem. Long-term abuse can permanently throw off the hypothalamic feedback system, which is needed in order to monitor the amount of HGH produced by the pituitary gland. This results in a hindrance of the body's natural production of HGH, and therefore speeds up the entire aging process.

The Discovery of HGH

HGH was first isolated in 1956 and identified as a chemical compound composed of a 191 amino acid chain. Attempts at isolation were performed in order to develop a treatment to aid a child's growth in the event that it had been stunted. At this point, HGH was only able to be obtained from human pituitary glands. The extraction process was expensive and time consuming, and there were problems with purification. However, in 1985, Nobel-prize winning scientist, Herbert Boyer, who aided in the development of genetic engineering, hired scientist David Goeddel to genetically engineer HGH. They were successful due to the recently acquired ability of scientists to splice genes and clone proteins. Soon after their success of making a recombinant (lab made) form of HGH, another company followed with their own HGH that was one amino acid closer to the human body. According to the Orphan Drug Act passed by Congress around that time, both companies could own market share for this recombinant HGH for 7 years. A patented, bio-engineered form of HGH could finally be easily manufactured in large quantities for the growth hormone-deficient children in the United States.

Shortly after this, however, it became clear that the main potential of this new recombinant HGH was with the aging population. HGH was eventually approved by the FDA for use in human experiments. This allowed scientist to work with it more in an anti-aging capacity. Dr. Daniel Rudman, from the Medical College of Wisconsin, published the results of his peer-reviewed, double-blind study utilizing HGH with the elderly in *The New England Journal of Medicine* (July 1990). His premise: If hormonal levels control the aging process, replacing these hormones should reverse it substantially! He proved this theory with flying colors in this study which laid the groundwork for scientists all over the world to look at HGH replacement to possibly treat aging and all its related diseases.

It is hard to measure an increase in someone's HGH levels because it is secreted in pulses. However, it is easy to measure increases in IGF-1 levels (a hormone similar to insulin in that it plays an important role in growth in childhood and adulthood), which has a direct connection to increases in HGH. There is a larger study on HGH to date: The Chein Study in Palm Springs Life Extension Institute—involved 202 patients and was done after Dr. Chein had completed work with over 800 patients from 1994-1996. His results were favorable in that they brought HGH levels back to the levels that would be found in a twenty-year-old, and this was done so by specifically raising the IGF-1 factors. Additionally, there was nothing indicative of cancer, and there were even a few decreases in factors that are monitored for the probability of prostate cancer (no testosterone used). These results are consistent with most studies on HGH injection results. There are more than 28,000 written studies world-wide reporting positive results with the use of HGH.

In spite of all this, there were still those who felt this type of hormone replacement therapy was unsafe. This fear was based on the fact that HGH could possibly spark unknown cancer cells in the body to "grow" or undiagnosed tumors to enlarge due to its "growth factor" aspect. This however, was never validated in any studies with HGH. Other possible side effects disputed were retention of fluids, joint pain, increased blood pressure, or "insulin resistance." It was also cost prohibitive, so this type of "replacement therapy" seemed vain at best and dangerous at worst.

Nevertheless, the research on HGH continued. As a result of the Chein study, as well as other studies, Stanford University medical researchers concluded in 1992 that it was possible that physiological HGH replacement might reverse or prevent some of the inevitable signs of aging.

Dr. Chein pioneered the use of the low-dose/high-frequency method of giving HGH, as this was discovered to have fewer, minor side effects, such as swelling, edema, and carpal tunnel syndrome. This method laid the groundwork for the less invasive homeopathic use of HGH, which administers small doses over time in a diluted form so that there are no documented side effects. For a better understanding of homeopathic medicine refer to Appendix G. Most people report similar results from taking homeopathic HGH as those taking injectable HGH. In my center, I advocate the use of a homeopathic blend of HGH over injectable HGH. (Refer to Chapter 8).

Howard Turney is often named by the media as the "Father of Growth Hormone" because he was responsible for creating the first anti-aging clinic in Mexico with HGH as a primary therapy. He has dedicated his life to promoting HGH as an anti-aging modality. He himself states that he had used injectable HGH for over eight years but has now switched to the homeopathic form. At present, he is advocating homeopathic HGH to those who contact him.

Using Homeopathic HGH

Medical studies show that small amounts of HGH taken frequently works better than large doses taken less frequently by injection (Howard, 1998, p. 22).

The spectacular results that we had seen with homeopathic hCG, as opposed to injectable hCG, for weight loss were what motivated me to determine if the homeopathic form of HGH was also a viable replacement for injectable HGH due to cost and safety factors. What we discovered was, while results are not as quick, we consistently note improvements in our clients who use it faithfully. Homeopathic blends of HGH are reported to produce about sixty to eighty percent of the results achieved with injectable HGH. Homeopathic medicine gently works to rebalance the body. Furthermore, it does not force the body in any one direction, as prescription drugs do. By working with the physics of the body (energy), not the chemistry, there are no documented chemical side effects. Homeopathic HGH can be used in combination with almost any medication. Unfortunately, the medical community does not yet accept homeopathic medicine as being valid; therefore, this method for administering HGH is not promoted to the public. Nonetheless, many Hollywood stars use homeopathic HGH for its skin-beautifying benefits while many professional athletes use it for improved performance.

The Many Benefits of HGH

When HGH is supplemented, benefits include more muscle mass in relation to body fat, equaling a better muscle-to-fat ratio. This is due in part to cells becoming less "insulin resistant," which will lower blood sugar levels and increase the body's fat-burning ability. When this is enhanced by any type of resistance training, there tends to be quick gains in muscle strength, size, and tone as well. This improved muscle-to-fat ratio will always result in improved overall weight management.

HGH's role in protein metabolism enhances the movement of amino acids through the cell membranes into the cell, enhances the cell's ability to synthesize and create proteins, and causes a decrease in the breakdown of cellular protein for energy. Proper protein metabolism is key to looking and feeling youthful.

When it comes to skin changes while taking HGH, studies show increased elasticity in skin, better texture of skin, and the ability for skin tissue to hold water (babies hold ninety percent water while adults and the elderly go down to levels as low as forty percent). HGH has an effect on hair as well. New hair growth can occur, hair loss is often halted, and some color can return to gray hair over time.

Regarding women's health, supplemental HGH can result in menstrual cycle regulation, decreased hot flashes, increased libido and an overall zest for life. In men, HGH has been known to aid with erectile dysfunction. The benefits for both sexes may include increased energy, better mood, emotional stability, improved memory, increased flexibility, decreased bone loss with age, decreased cholesterol and triglyceride levels, faster healing of injuries, quicker recovery, resistance to common illness, and increased hydration of the body (it allows for a better ability to hold water in the tissues, similarly to that of a twenty year old). Some people also report improvements in eyesight.

NOTE: These changes happen over a period of one to six months. However, the first thing that you will notice, which will prove the effectiveness, is your sleep will be uninterrupted and very deep and you will wake up refreshed in the morning.

Benefits of Homeopathic HGH over Injectable HGH

1. The homeopathic form of HGH is safer. Any side effects with homeopathic substances are extremely rare and there are virtually no drug interactions either. There have been no documented drug reactions with homeopathic HGH.

2. The homeopathic form of HGH is easy to use. Spray or drop under the tongue daily; no injections are required.

3. The homeopathic form of HGH is less expensive than the injectable HGH which can run up to $1,000 a month.

4. The homeopathic form of HGH uses low doses with higher frequency which has been proven by studies to be the best method of dosing for HGH.

5. The homeopathic form of HGH gently encourages the pituitary gland to release and supplement the body's natural HGH, which has decreased with time. This means it aids the body in achieving balance or homeostasis.

Know What You Are Buying

There has been some controversy over the use of HGH in certain forms (oral dosing) and the fact that some products on the market do not really contain any HGH. Molecularly, HGH is very large and it cannot be absorbed sublingually (under the tongue) nor can it be assimilated through the digestive system. So it is easy to understand why its sale in an ineffective form would be questioned. As stated, there are only two ways of getting effective results using HGH. If you decide to use HGH, make sure that it is either 1) real injectable HGH, which requires a doctor's prescription or 2) a true homeopathic HGH. If you see "homeopathic-like" on the label, it is not a true homeopathic formula.

Putting HGH into a Larger Protocol for Best Results

Another area of confusion is that many advertisers "promise people the world" from just taking a supplement without some lifestyle changes. Exaggerated claims about HGH products are out there and companies can make it seem like their product is the only answer. Any supplement becomes more effective with a few healthy lifestyle adjustments. Therefore, my center's protocol for using our homeopathic HGH is more than just taking the homeopathic drops. I encourage my clients to take steps towards greater health by what they do, not just what they take (pills, drops, supplements, and so on). Once they lose weight on the protocol offered at my health center, I often suggest they get involved in strength training along with using homeopathic HGH. This supplement will then allow for faster muscle growth and tone which can be very motivating.

To get the best results from HGH, I suggest the following lifestyle changes:

1. Engage in daily stress management to reduce cortisol production, including all of the strategies mentioned throughout this book, such as meditation, adequate sleep, "sound-wave" therapy, and so on. Excess stress hormones, like cortisol, naturally suppress or inhibit HGH production and speeds aging in the body. (Read more in Chapter 8).

2. Make an effort to keep your sex hormones balanced as well. (Read more in Chapter 2 and Chapter 5). This offers a better foundation to get faster results with HGH. I personally recommend that women use a "trans-dermal" progesterone cream and address existing adrenal issues before using HGH (mentioned in Chapter 8). HGH can then seem to take them to "the next level" physically. Natural hormone balancing of estrogen and progesterone will eliminate most of the bothersome symptoms, but HGH can then take energy higher, increase libido, and put the finishing touches on appearance (skin, hair and muscle to fat ratio as mentioned).

3. Get some daily movement to dispel stress and engage in resistance training two to three times per week. There are many options available for you to choose from. As we age, if we do not tend to our bodies, we lose one percent of our muscle per year (which translates to an alarming ten percent per decade). Once you have achieved times in a ten-day period will be adequate to maintain that level.

4. Decrease your intake of refined carbohydrates (white sugar and white flour). Keep your consumption to a minimum of one to two servings per day, if any.

5. Get adequate sleep. Aim for deep restorative sleep every night of at least eight hours. This deeper sleep will happen on HGH, but you must provide the time and restful place so that it can. Also, be sure your room is as dark as possible to facilitate adequate melatonin (sleep hormone) production. Covering up the bright red numbers on your alarm clock that usually shine in your face can really help!

Your health is not something handed to you in a bottle. It is a co- created process in which you voluntarily take part. It requires, on a physical level, that you give your body the nutrients it needs, while removing harmful toxins. Mental "shift s" in how you perceive aging are vital as well. Truly having the "anti-aging" mindset will reduce stress on the central nervous system and is the key to keeping all hormones balanced. You can implement this mindset by . . .

. . . loving yourself and others
. . . always wanting to grow
. . . never limiting your potential based on an "age"
. . . always forgiving, letting go of past hurts, guilt and anger
. . . connecting to a higher source and then radiating out that love and energy to all those around you

Most women look at aging negatively, and this is understandably a popular train of thought, especially if you feel like you are "losing" your youth. I feel it would be much better to see and appreciate what you gain as you age. Knowledge and experience grow with age but so can wisdom and deeper truth if you pursue it. If you can keep your health intact, then you can have the healthy body of your youth in addition to the knowledge and wisdom that only comes with years and experience. You can stay healthy and have vitality as you age by incorporating good nutrition, exercise, meditation, a positive outlook, and proper supplementation (like HGH)!

There are those rare people who age beautifully and I let them be my guide on life's journey. I have such a friend, who is now 80 years old and she truly is a wise and beautiful soul. I let this example inspire me. In saying that, let me leave you with the mindset I strive to have when I think of myself moving along with "Father Time" . . . I finally realized that he can be my friend.

As I age, I wish to become more translucent to the light that is in me . . . not to thicken and harden up with a callused soul, but to be free flowing, flexible, and transparent to the power inside me . . . to let others see it and marvel . . . to be a link in connecting collective souls not a wedge between people just taking up space . . .

They will not see my wrinkles, *they will see my light*

The will not feel my pain, *but feel my warmth*

They will not hear my complaints, *but absorb my joy*

I will not touch them in passing, *but will touch their life for the better*

They will breathe in my energy and it will energize them, ease fear, offer hope . . . that the place they can go (wisdom) is much better than where they have been (youth) . . .

CHAPTER 8

Specific Solutions to the Hormone Shift

What if . . .
. . . you liked the body you saw reflecting back at you in the mirror?
. . . you felt energetic, slept deeper, and could go off your medication?
. . . you could improve your relationships and "spark" with your partner?
. . . you had the confidence to do something you always wanted to do?
What if . . . you could become all you were meant to be?

It is not a dream; I see it happen every day. When women achieve hormonal balance, balance in their life soon follows as well! Can you imagine how you will feel when you see your life improve and the lives of those around you improve as a result? Everything can improve; including your job, your relationships, your skills, your spirituality . . . all of it! You can like how you look and feel, and you can lead a healthy lifestyle when you find your perfect hormonal balance. The feelings of being burdened by extra weight or feeling tired, depressed or anxious can dissipate faster than you may think when your hormones become balanced. Negative feelings are certainly not going to further you down the road to better intimacy, improved parenting, and increased job productivity. Low self-esteem, as a result of these feelings, is definitely not guiding you along the path of self actualization and deeper self-awareness. All of this can come to an end. When your hormones are balanced you have the foundation to think more clearly and you have the motivation to make better decisions leading to a healthier you—physically, mentally, emotionally and spiritually! With this exciting discovery in mind, let's get started going over the specifics of how you can do this.

You now have a basic understanding of the interaction between sex and stress hormones and the balance that the body strives to achieve. Simply stated, the underlying cause of your symptoms—whether it is PMS, low thyroid, hot flashes, stubborn weight, depression, or rapid aging—is all connected to a simple hormonal imbalance. By now I am sure this concept resonates with you.

Now that a foundation has been set for what needs to be done, I would like to tell you a little more specifically about what you can do to naturally solve these hormonal problems. I have categorized the basic symptoms into a flow chart (Figure 8-1) and will direct you to the solution that will best suit your specific needs. Later in the chapter we will review in detail each of these three simple, safe and fast-acting solutions to help you look and feel your best (Sections #1-3). Finally, I will present an optional solution (Section#4) that will enhance any of the initial three you may have chosen to fit your needs.

To determine the solution(s) for you, first decide if weight is an issue with your other hormonal symptoms or if weight is not an issue and you just have basic PMS and menopausal hormonal symptoms. It would be rare to have any of the weight-related issues listed and not suffer from some basic PMS and menopausal symptoms which are caused by "estrogen dominance." Issues with weight typically go hand-in-hand with this imbalance as a woman moves on in years. For the purpose of this chart, we will consider your weight issue to be due to a hormone imbalance and proceed with you choosing your solution based on the need for weight loss.

Figure 8-1
Natural Solutions to the Hormone Shift

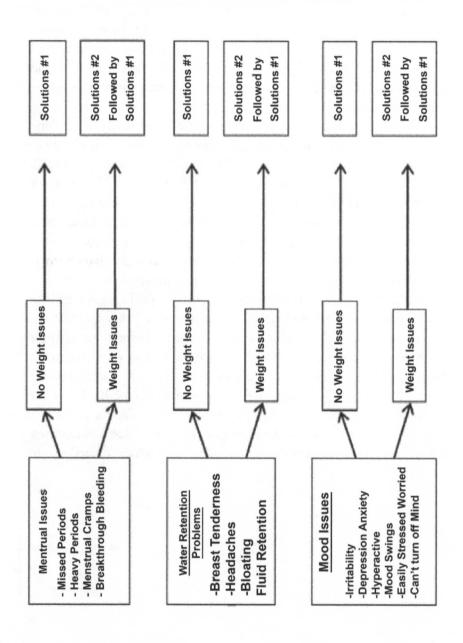

Figure 8-1 (continued) Natural Solutions to the Hormone Shift

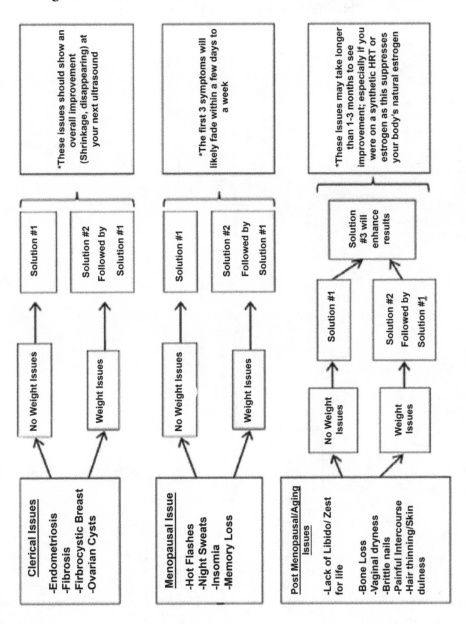

Figure 8-1 (continued)
Natural Solutions to the Hormone Shift

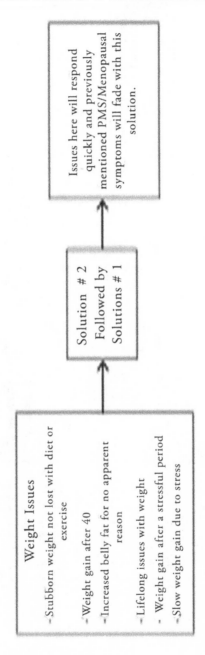

Weight Issues

- Stubborn weight not lost with diet or exercise
- Weight gain after 40
- Increased belly fat for no apparent reason
- Lifelong issues with weight
- Weight gain after a stressful period
- Slow weight gain due to stress

Solution # 2 Followed by Solutions # 1

Issues here will respond quickly and previously mentioned PMS/Menopausal symptoms will fade with this solution.

Benefits of Natural Solutions for the Hormone Shift

The real benefit that lies in naturally working with the body is just that, you are working with the body to establish balance. This is what the body naturally strives to accomplish—a state of homeostasis. The natural supplements that I am about to recommend support the body in its own healing process. They do not impede healing by taxing the liver or the immune or digestive systems. These supplements support the entire balance of the endocrine system by focusing on adrenal fatigue/ exhaustion and offering building blocks for the body to make what it needs for daily stressful challenges. The next step is to build the body's reserves of the necessary hormonal precursors (substances from which hormones are made), while also supplying the main deficient hormone, progesterone (shown in Solution #1), or by supplying the body with the ability to make it (shown in Solution #2). This will establish the much needed balance of progesterone and estrogen.

Side Effects of Natural Solutions

When working with natural solutions, the health risks and side effects are extremely rare and minimal. I phrase it as, "There are no documented side effects." However, in each applicable section, a few rare but possible occurrences will be mentioned. These are simply observations that may seem quite insignificant, short-term and minimally inconvenient but I wanted to bring them to your attention nonetheless. There is really no comparison between these minor, rare occurrences and side effects of medications and surgeries. It is always wise to work with an experienced health professional to guide you through any issues you may encounter.

Precautions with Natural Solutions

Precautions, like side effects, are minimal with these mentioned natural remedies due to the fact that homeopathic medicine and natural hormones (or hormone precursors) do not tend to interact with traditional medication, which you may be taking when you start a natural regimen. The biggest precaution with some medications is that

143

as the body stabilizes (often quickly), medications need to be reduced to parallel this balance or you are at risk for being over medicated. These medication modifications will be mentioned specifically with any recommended "solution" to which they apply.

The *under use* of the recommended natural supplements will result in achieving inadequate results—whereas *over use* will not be overly problematic, except for the cost of the wasted product. This means that you cannot overdose with these natural solutions unlike prescription medication.

The above statement does not, however, apply to other natural and valid supplements that utilize herbs. Some herbs can interact with medications and too much of an herb can cause complications in the body. Even though this may be rare, I want to bring it to your attention and distinguish herbal remedies from homeopathic supplementation and natural hormone creams, which I will be describing in the solutions below. Although herbs are natural, it is still wise to work closely with an herbalist and let your doctor know of all the herbs that you are taking. They will be able to instruct you better on which medications these herbs may possibly interact with.

Solutions to the Hormone Shift

These options offer you the ability to balance hormones for improved weight, mood, and health all while restoring your youthful vitality!

Section 1: Use **"Solution #1"** if you want to balance your hormones and get rid of PMS and menopausal symptoms when **NO weight loss is needed** (or only five to seven pounds). This solution can be used along with your own diet for improved results. You then have the option to look at adding Solution #3 as a finishing touch at any time.

Section 2: Use **"Solution #2"** if you want to lose weight (especially in your most stubborn areas) as well as reset your metabolism, balance your hormones, get rid of PMS and eliminate menopausal symptoms. This will run thirty, sixty or ninety days depending on how much weight you want to lose. A certain overall hormonal balance is achieved in one thirty day round. Then it is important to stabilize or anchor your new hormone balance with Solution #1 on a daily basis. You always have the option to look at adding Solution #3 as a finishing touch or during your weight loss rounds at anytime.

Section 3: Use **"Solution #3"** (Optional) as a finishing touch after Solution #2 or with Solution #1 to slow signs of aging and improve the skin and muscle tone or to deepen sleep to aid in repairing the body. If weight is not an issue, it is best that you at least do Solution #1 for about two to four weeks as a foundation before adding in Solution #3. This will allow your sex hormones to be balanced which enhances Solution #3.

Section 4: Using the information in Section 4—which describes an overall solution to all hormonal imbalances—will enhance Solutions #1-3 dramatically. This is due to stress being the main culprit in the hormonal Shift to begin with. I hope you will read and apply this information as well.

Section 1

Solution #1 Natural Hormone Therapy for the Hormone Shift . . .
relieving symptoms of PMS and Menopause

After reading Chapter 1, The Hormone Shift & How it Affects Your Body, it is evident that you need to work with your progesterone levels in order to balance out your estrogen. This balance eliminates PMS and menopausal symptoms, which all stem from "estrogen dominance." Also, addressing your stress levels, and the subsequent adrenal fatigue/exhaustion that accompanies chronic stress, will be an important factor for achieving the necessary progesterone levels. If progesterone is administered, but stress is still chronic, progesterone will be drained again as it will get converted into cortisol. In this case, the symptoms will not permanently disappear. However, when adrenal fatigue/exhaustion is addressed with supplemental support for the adrenal gland, the progesterone therapy will be much more effective. Let's look at how to do that. Please keep in mind the basics of what you read in Chapter 2 (The Hormone Shift & Menopause). Even if you are over the age of 50, through menopause and have some symptoms of low estrogen (vaginal dryness, bone loss, dry skin, low libido), extra estrogen most often is not necessary because your skin and fat stores are able to produce estrone (the weaker estrogen). Due to its risks, my suggestion is to try the natural hormone creams, to be discussed below, before adding any additional estrogen to your body.

The effect of Solution #1 on a pre-menopausal woman or a postmenopausal woman can be seen in Figure 8 -2. Even though the way to resolve the hormonal imbalance is the same (progesterone therapy and adrenal support), the end result is catered to the woman's need in her particular stage of life. This is due to the body using these natural supplements to balance itself!

Figure 8-2 Premenopausal Woman's Solution:

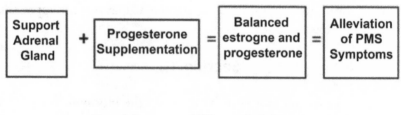

Post Menopausal Woman's Solution:

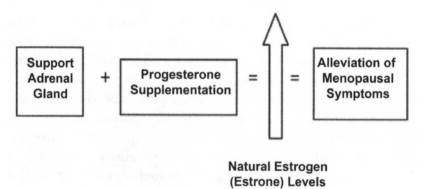

**Natural Estrogen
(Estrone) Levels**

Let us start with progesterone supplementation in order to raise your levels of this needed hormone to balance out "estrogen dominance." This can be done gently, naturally and safely. The balance between estrogen and progesterone will help you feel calmer immediately, and as depression lifts, sleep is deeper and vitality returns. Over the course of one month you should start to notice your PMS symptoms diminish as your next cycle comes and over the following two months, the more clinical symptoms of "estrogen dominance" like fibroids, fibrocystic breasts, and endometriosis, can begin to diminish. Potential surgeries for these conditions will often be avoided. In this balanced hormonal state, you are in a much better position to be able to burn extra body fat, reduce fluid retention, and have optimal mood and motivation for making healthy food choices and the energy needed for exercise. In short, proper hormone balance promotes healthy lifestyle choices.

Ways to Supplement with Progesterone:

1. Oral progesterone supplements are almost always synthetic. Synthetic forms of progesterone are called "progestin" and these synthetic substitutes do not have the same qualities of real progesterone (read more in Chapter 5). Some oral forms of progesterone are natural but there are still other issues with this form of progesterone supplementation. Overall, massive dosages are required (200 mg) and administered due to poor absorption through the digestive system. The high dosages are sometimes ten times the amount of progesterone the body produces naturally (about 20 mg per day) but are necessary because they are poorly absorbed. It is sad to say but because the majority of our population has poor digestion, optimal amounts of any oral supplementation—even some prescription drugs—are not utilized as well as they could be. It is often not known exactly how much (dosage) is getting into your system. In addition, oral forms of progesterone need to pass through the liver, which is often already overtaxed with environmental and daily toxins. Therefore, I do not suggest this form of progesterone therapy.

2. Sublingual progesterone supplementation, which is administered by placement under the tongue and easily absorbed due to it bypassing the digestive system. Sublingual progesterone is often prescribed by doctors and filled by pharmacists when a

bio-identical model of hormone therapy is used (see Chapter 2). While this method is prescribed less often than cream forms, I believe it is becoming more common and is a viable option if you opt to use the bio-identical model of hormone therapy. This is due to the fact that some of the bio-identical cream forms of progesterone do not go directly into the bloodstream (more to come on this) and build up in the fatty tissue causing overloads of this hormone in the body. This tends to cause all PMS and menopausal symptoms you were trying to eliminate to suddenly return.

3. <u>Cream-based progesterone</u> supplementation is a simple, efficient and effective way to augment your natural progesterone levels and it is available without a prescription. The cream can be applied to designated areas of the body once or twice a day as instructed. Cream-based progesterone is what I suggest to my clients and utilize at my health center. I will explain below how to be sure your progesterone cream will not build up in your fatty tissue.

What to look for in a progesterone cream:

1. Look for a progesterone cream that is a USP Progesterone. The term USP refers to the grade or purity of the product and is the shortened form of the term *United States Pharmacopeia*. This is a more standardized form; therefore, a higher quality. It should be listed on the label this way.

2. Look for progesterone cream with other ingredients that support the entire endocrine (female) system. An example would be ingredients such as DHEA and/or pregnenolone (mentioned in Chapter 1). These two master hormones can be used by the body as "building blocks," to aid in the production of sex hormones, such as estrogen and testosterone if they are ever low. This is a much more conservative and safe approach than directly administering these two "more risky" hormones directly to the body as done in the bio-identical model of hormone replacement therapy.

3. Another example of a type of supportive ingredient in a progesterone cream is Maca root, which has been used for centuries in South America. It acts on the hypothalamus and pituitary glands to produce precursors to female hormones so the body can build them as needed. Maca root also positively affects an overworked adrenal gland, and therefore supports the endocrine system in a regulatory manner. It is always best to use a progesterone cream that offers additional endocrine support so the body has additional tools to balance itself.

4. Look for a progesterone cream with a true "trans-dermal" delivery system. The major advantage of a "trans-dermal" delivery system is that the active ingredient bypasses the digestive system for quicker and more efficient delivery. Unlike a lot of prescription drugs, a "trans-dermal" approach also puts less stress on the liver. Another advantage is that progesterone cream with a true "trans-dermal" delivery system will not allow buildup of the hormone in the body because it is delivered directly into the bloodstream and then clears out within eighteen to twenty-four hours. This is very similar to how water-soluble vitamins B and C are flushed out of the system if taken in excess. "Trans-dermal" creams work through the use of liposomes*. These creams do not have to be rotated in their application points, even when used daily, and they are applied to thin skinned areas like the inner arms, neck and upper chest or back of the knees to allow quick penetration.

*Microscopic membrane-formed sacs, often from naturally- derived phospholipids; used to allow special molecular ingredients to be able to bypass the barrier of the skin and get into the bloodstream.

Liposomes are often used in high level skincare and by drug companies i.e.Nicoderm patch as well as the estrogen patch. Experienced chemists use liposomes in prescription drugs and natural supplements to allow for quick absorption into the bloodstream. The chemist who formulated the natural hormone creams that we utilize at my center, *Kyle Holderman of Endoderm Labratories Inc.*, stated, "A 'trans-dermal' delivery system is a vital key in the effectiveness of hormone balancing creams. Liposomes can encapsulate the molecules of the effective ingredients to allow them to travel down past the natural skin barrier to the bloodstream where they can be effectively used by the body."

Northern Lipids Inc., A contract research organization that provides products and services to biotechnology companies that are engaged in the development of pharmaceutical products, states on their website that "Lipid-based 'trans-dermal' delivery systems are an accepted, proven, commercially viable strategy to formulate pharmaceuticals, for topical, oral, pulmonary or parenteral delivery."

If the directions accompanying a hormone cream instruct you to apply it to fatty areas of the body and instruct you to rotate the application areas, this shows that the delivery system is not truly "trans-dermal." This application rotation is to help avoid buildup. Most of these types of creams will also contain an alcohol base, which is another clear indication that the cream is not a true "trans- dermal" delivery system. Fatty tissue can only hold a certain amount of progesterone, or any other hormone, and after months of use, the progesterone will build up to the point of saturation. Upon saturation, the body can experience a high rise in progesterone levels, as evidenced by a saliva test, causing all hormonal-related symptoms to return. Again, this is due to the principle that too much of something in the body is the same as not enough. Be aware of the delivery system for the natural progesterone cream that you choose because it, as stated above, makes a big difference.

When women have come to my center feeling terrible, and their saliva test showed very high levels of progesterone, it was an indicator that the progesterone cream they were using did not have a "trans-dermal" delivery system. I observed that the creams they were using had a less effective alcohol-based delivery system. These creams were either purchased from a health food store or were bio-identical in form, having been prescribed by an overzealous doctor. In my experience, doctors following the bio-identical model will sometimes use creams that have a poor delivery system, coupled with a high dosage, and then never re-test their patients' hormone levels. Remember, too much progesterone can yield the same symptoms as low progesterone— bringing back all original PMS or menopausal symptoms caused by "estrogen dominance." High progesterone in the body can only occur as a result of product buildup over time in the fatty tissues of the body.

This very thing happened to my own mother after menopause! Due to the menopausal symptoms that she was experiencing, she decided to go to a local apothecary and meet with an educated pharmacist to check her hormone levels.

Unfortunately, she decided to take this route instead of working with me because her insurance covered this type of pharmacy prescribed bio-identical hormone therapy. After having saliva tests, it was found that her progesterone levels were low and she was put on a progesterone cream. Initially, she did well and all of her symptoms from her "estrogen dominance" went away. After six to seven months of this therapy, she began to feel depressed, anxious, unable to sleep, and her heart would race at times. During this time, which was eight years ago, frequent saliva testing was not the norm; therefore, after hearing her complaints, the pharmacist said that she should not worry. These seemingly minor symptoms were later followed by heart-attack like symptoms to which I responded by taking her to the emergency room. The doctors could not find anything wrong with her heart. When she got out of the hospital the next day, she decided to insist on another hormone saliva test. When tested, her progesterone levels were sky high compared to her original saliva test. She was clearly experiencing a buildup of progesterone in her fatty tissue. Too much progesterone that is built up in the body will often cause the progesterone receptor sites to "burn out," rendering it unable to do its intended job. This can cause an over stimulatory effect by the estrogen in the body (now unopposed by the ineffective progesterone) which can even adversely affect the heart.

My colleague and I advised her to discontinue the hormone cream prescribed by the pharmacist. After a few months, her progesterone had returned to relatively normal levels and she felt much better. We then administered the natural progesterone cream that I use in my center, for one month. After which we retested her progesterone levels and they finally showed within normal range. Furthermore, her initial symptoms of "estrogen dominance" that had returned, disappeared again. We continued to test regularly, and her levels remained normal. Although the pharmacy refunded the money that my mother had spent on their cream, they never admitted that they had mishandled her care.

Remember, high levels of progesterone are never found naturally in the body. In American women, levels of this hormone are usually low unless there is a buildup. If you do supplement with progesterone cream and are showing elevated levels of progesterone, check to see if your cream has a "trans-dermal" delivery system. With a true "trans-dermal" delivery system, any excess of product or ingredients should simply be excreted during urination and never cause a buildup in the body.

The natural "trans-dermal" progesterone cream that I use in my center fits all of the above criteria mentioned and is called **Pro Plus**. It is available at your local BeBalanced Center with a simple symptom-based questionnaire that you can print out. This will provide easy and effective dosage recommendations based on the symptoms that you are experiencing.

Now that you understand how to most efficiently and safely administer progesterone, we need to address your adrenal fatigue/exhaustion that is actually at the core of your hormonal imbalance. As mentioned earlier, your daily stress must be taken into consideration anytime that you wish to increase your progesterone levels. If you are losing progesterone through its conversion to cortisol, then it defeats the purpose. A few things need to happen to address this issue. Locate the causes of stress in your life (see Chapter 1), and then come up with a plan to lower these factors—for example more sleep, physical therapy, chiropractic care, or even less processed foods. This may take some thought and time, but it will aid in balancing your hormones (Section #4 will offer a great practical solution). In turn, your overall quality of life will improve, the aging process will slow, and you are better protected against certain diseases.

The fact remains, however, you can only—or *will only*—change your lifestyle so much to reduce your stress levels. Therefore, taking supplements to support the adrenal gland is essential to this process. Supplements that get depleted when we are under stress (such as vitamins B and C) as well as the hormone DHEA and/or pregnenolone, which also support the adrenal gland, will help. I have observed that many herbs, even administered by master herbalists, commonly offer minimal results. Some herbs do offer benefits but they take a long time to become effective, can be expensive, and need to be monitored closely because of possible drug interactions. Additionally, client/ patient adherence is low because of the slow results. These supplements and herbs are also administered orally, and have to go through the digestive system.

Typically, at the point at which a woman needs this supplementation, her digestive system is already weakened and therefore the oral supplements are not effectively absorbed. So, let us return to the idea of allowing the body to absorb effective ingredients through the skin which is much more efficient. In my practice, I have found that it is beneficial to aid the body in making the cortisol that it requires daily without the need to steal the newly supplemented progesterone. This can be done with daily use of a stress-relieving, natural hormone support cream called **Soothe Stress** that supports the adrenal gland. This natural "transdermal" hormone cream gives the body the building blocks that it needs to manufacture cortisol so that progesterone levels can be increased to attain balance faster, yielding better symptom cessation. **Soothe Stress** contains the master hormones pregnenolone and DHEA. It is now known that DHEA aids the overall metabolism but it also allows the body to rebalance so it can manufacture estrogen and testosterone as it deems necessary. A much safer approach to hormone therapy is to let the body make estrogen and testosterone as needed. This is in contrast to traditional HRT and bio-identical hormone replacement that tend to prescribe estrogen and testosterone to women showing low levels on their saliva tests. The risk of overdose is increased when supplementing with these two hormones that have not been proven safe long term. Therefore, it is usually best to allow the body to make what it needs by supplementing it with master hormones.

The main purpose of this book is not to simply promote supplements but to provide hormone education so you can make informed decisions. However, when it comes to adrenal support, I would be remiss to not highlight the cream we use called Soothe Stress. Our chemist came up with this formula and I have seen nothing like it on the market yet. For my clients, I pair **Soothe Stress** with natural progesterone cream. This provides tremendous synergistic results as they tend to work together toward perfect balance. When the adrenal gland is supported in this manner and progesterone levels rise through supplementation; oftentimes, common menopausal symptoms like hot flashes diminish within a week or two. The only precaution with **Soothe Stress** is that depending on the state of your adrenal gland, whether it be fatigued or fully exhausted, it is best to avoid application close to bedtime. I make this recommendation because it can provide additional energy, which might keep you awake. Also, if too much of the product is applied at one time, it can give a "coffee high" feeling for an hour or so, which may not be desirable. Lastly, there is a rare chance that low energy can be a result for a few days as the body is using this cream to repair your adrenal gland. The low energy is an indication of the body's need to rest. These few minor possibilities are negligible in comparison to the side effects from prescription drugs. The overall benefits of the **Soothe Stress** cream, coupled with fast results, make these possible inconveniences completely worthwhile. I have thousands of clients who swear by this efficient method of supporting adrenal health. **Soothe Stress** is at your local BeBalanced Center. It too is accompanied with a simple symptom-based questionnaire that will provide easy dosage recommendations.

As the stress cycle in the body is broken and your overall stress is lowered, the **Soothe Stress** cream dosage can typically be reduced or even eliminated. Additionally, the progesterone cream can be lowered to minute amounts, which makes it cost-effective long term. Even at the lowest dosage it will help keep hormone levels in the safe and optimal range (See dosage recommendations below).

Because the chance for hormonal buildup is nonexistent, it is not necessary to pre-test your hormone levels before using **Pro Plus** or **Soothe Stress**. You can simply take the symptom-based questionnaire at the end of Chapter 1 to determine your level of "estrogen dominance." Whatever stage of the shift you find yourself in, getting your adrenal fatigue/ exhaustion under control will help to better manage efficient cortisol production. Furthermore, supplementing with natural progesterone is a conservative, but effective means to balancing your hormones. Your body knows best. It will work toward reaching and maintaining homeostasis; the perfect balance.

Dosage of Progesterone Cream

Generally, a safe dosage for progesterone cream mimics the body's own production. The dosing instructions I use are based on Dr. Lee's recommendations. Additionally, the **Soothe Stress** cream for adrenal support or any preferred method of adrenal support can also be used to "preserve" the added progesterone and keep it from being converted into cortisol. Again, this vital step is essential but rarely taken into account by doctors or healthcare practitioners when giving progesterone for symptoms of "estrogen dominance."

Remember, progesterone delivered through a cream is not going to harm your body or cause symptoms like that of too much estrogen. If you are using a completely "trans-dermal" approach, hormone buildup will not be an issue nor will "overdosing" at any one time of application.

According to Dr. Lee (2006) in *Hormone Balance Made Simple*, the body produces about 20 mg of progesterone per day (p. 123). This amount is typically equal to about a half teaspoon, but I still advise that you check the label on your product for specific information. For example, the **Pro Plus** cream is one quarter teaspoon for a 20 mg dose. The progesterone cream (if in a "trans-dermal" delivery) should be applied to thin-skinned areas like the inner arms, neck and upper chest, back of knees or even bottom of the feet. For a younger pre-menopausal woman, who is still menstruating but suffers from PMS, 20 mg once a day, on days fourteen through twenty-eight of her cycle or until the onset of her period, would probably be suitable to start. This timing mimics the body's way of making progesterone, which should rise in the luteal phase of the cycle—the second half of the cycle. If a higher dosage is needed to relieve symptoms, an increase to 20 mg twice a day might be in order. This would be applied in the morning and then in the evening. For a peri-menopausal or menopausal woman the progesterone cream can be applied daily then stopped after twenty-five days for the four to five days of menstruation. For a postmenopausal woman who no longer gets a menstrual period, the cream can still be stopped for those four to five days to mimic a natural cycle. In this case, the 20 mg dosage used once or twice a day is administered until all symptoms are relieved. This can then be cut back to the minimal dosage needed to keep symptoms from returning. This conserves the product and is more cost-effective.

Your individual health-care professional can guide you on how much of the cream to use, but your symptoms should always be taken into account. If your symptoms do not subside, which means you have not yet achieved balance, the dosage either needs to be adjusted or the product/ delivery system is not working adequately. What I like about the **Pro Plus** and **Soothe Stress** creams is that all I need is a basic protocol for our women through the use of the mentioned questionnaire. The dosage can then be lowered or adjusted based on symptom relief without dangerous side effects.

Staying on progesterone therapy may be something you choose to do for the rest of your life. Think of it as a multivitamin for your hormones as part of a healthy lifestyle, which helps to keep you young. If you want to keep your hormones at a youthful level, even in your later years, be sure to keep your overall stress levels down, support your adrenal gland with some supplementation, and supplement with natural progesterone. Keeping your progesterone levels in optimal range will encourage your body to match this balance with your own "risk-free" estrogen coming from other (non- ovarian) sources, such as your skin and fat. As the body ages, estrogen is required in order to keep the tissues supple, including the walls of the vagina, as well as to protect the heart and prevent bone loss. Optimal levels of progesterone will even keep the estrogen receptor sites more sensitive, even in the presence of low estrogen. Progesterone supplementation will allow the body to make estrone from the fat and skin cells as estradiol from the ovaries begins to deplete closer to menopause. This allows for a smooth transition into menopause without hot flashes or other upsetting symptoms. Progesterone supplementation will also offer some immediate relief to the postmenopausal woman as the body begins to produce estrone due to progesterone levels coming back into an optimal range.

In conclusion, doing your homework on the natural progesterone cream you choose to supplement with will allow you to feel comfortable with it. Even though the FDA and the medical community often raise the issue of the lack of dosage control or lack of clinical trials performed with natural supplements; hopefully, now you understand they are safe. In addition, Dr. Lee had pioneered research with progesterone therapy long ago proving it was safe for long-term use. The argument is also sometimes posed that these natural hormone creams cannot be properly monitored. This is a good point. Since most natural supplements do not have FDA approval, a wise consumer should thoroughly check ingredients and the source and reputation of the store, website, or healthcare provider from where the product is purchased. However, as we discussed earlier, when using a hormone cream with a true "trans-dermal" delivery system it is not necessary to monitor your dosage amounts. It should also be noted that natural supplements do not have to be closely monitored with lab testing since they do not have the potentially serious side effects associated with overdoses of bio-identical hormones or prescription drugs. A woman knows how she feels, and if all of her symptoms are relieved, then most likely a healthy balance has been restored. After all, we do not need to test women who feel great and are healthy and energetic, do we?

Section 2

Solution #2 Using a Low Calorie Ketogenic/Glandular
Protocol for Weight Gained During the Hormone Shift
. . . and relieving symptoms of PMS & Menopause

After reading Chapter 3 on the Hormone Shift & Weight, you are now aware of the use of glandulars with a lower calorie diet to induce a ketogenic state for effective and efficient weight loss. As a review, glandular therapies involve utilizing glands, organs or tissue from healthy animals to improve the function of the same glands/organs in the person using them, because they contain enzymes and cofactors that support balance in the body. The glandular type that you take will have an affinity for (or attraction to) your matching gland in your body and therefore will help repair that gland. Glandular tissue extracts come in pill form or homeopathic form for all the major glands of the body such as the hypothalamus, pituitary, adrenal, ovarian and thyroid gland. The key here is to obtain good, clean glandular tissue and to used them properly.

Glandulars are easy and safe to work with especially in small doses or in a homeopathic form, such as I recommend in what I call a "low calorie ketogenic/glandular weight loss protocol." You will experience fast fat loss and you will naturally be balancing your sex hormones. The ketogenic state and the glandular blend will raise progesterone levels in the body for the alleviation of most PMS and menopausal symptoms (see Figure 8-3).

Figure 8-3
Solution #2 Affect on Hormones and Weight

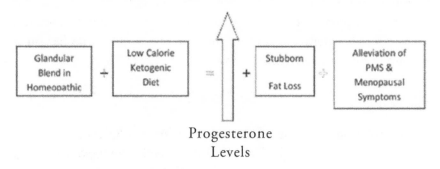

Progesterone
Levels

To get the best results, minimize any discomfort, and be able to sustain weight loss, there are some tips that I can provide. I strongly advocate that when using glandulars for weight loss, a low calorie ketogenic/glandular protocol consisting of an exact one-to-one ratio of carbohydrate to protein foods should be used, and done under professional guidance for best results. Similar to the use of herbs, using glandulars should come with some precautions. First of all, these are strong substances when used in pill or powder form that go to work directly on the cells of the body from a bio-chemistry perspective. All foods, vitamins, herbs, and medications work on the biology and the chemistry of the body. Just as with medications and herbs, glandulars in this form, when used in higher amounts, can over stimulate the body. This is especially true with adrenal and thyroid glandulars which can cause a hyper, feeling of panic that is not desirable. This is why I always prefer to use substances in a homeopathic form because homeopathic blends work on the physics of the body. This is a gentler way to nudge the body, or more specifically in this case, the glands, to perform optimally without over stimulating them. For more on how homeopathic blends work, see Appendix G.

I provide this guidance in my BeBalanced Center, or through my website, as we branch out to set up franchised BeBalanced Centers in other areas of the country (listed on the bebalancedcenters.com website). Working with a professional on your low calorie ketogenic/ glandular protocol is suggested. Even though homeopathic glandulars are safe for almost everyone, working with supervision will aid in helping you achieve optimal, lasting results. Remember, a low calorie ketogenic/ glandular protocol is short in length and provides fast results, but you still have to adjust your lifestyle for long-term health and weight maintenance.

We live in America in the twenty-first century, which is a far cry from the low-stress, less-toxic European lifestyle of sixty to seventy years ago, when a low calorie ketogenic protocol was initially introduced by Dr Simeons (using hCG). Today, some adjustments should be made to the overall process. Simply buying a homeopathic glandular blend from the Internet or a health food store will yield some fast results; however, these results do not last in comparison to the people who use homeopathic glandular blends with low a calorie ketogenic diet protocol. Only then can results be optimal and lasting, as it is part of a complete health program which addresses other stressors and health issues of the American lifestyle. In this process, it is essential that you make some easy lifestyle adjustments on the back end of the protocol. At BeBalanced Centers, we provide guidance and education that "anchors" women in their new hormonal balance after their initial weight loss.

Tips for using a low calorie ketogenic/glandular protocol for fat loss.

1. Homeopathic formulas can be used instead of pill or powder glandulars. From my own experience and observations, homeopathic glandular blends work as effectively or possibly more effectively than pill forms of glandulars, and are safer because homeopathic glandulars cannot over stimulate the body from a bio-chemistry perspective. Using your glandular in a homeopathic form prevents this, as homeopathy works with small amounts administered over a period of time, gently working with the energy or "physics" of the body.

2. Use an FDA-approved homeopathic manufacturer. I recommend choosing a homeopathic formula that comes from an FDA-approved laboratory. Even though the FDA does not state that homeopathy in general is effective; in FDA-approved labs, inspections are periodically done for quality control. This

ensures that the homeopathic formulas comply with current Good Manufacturing Practices (cGMPs) and the Code of Federal Regulations (CFRs). This protects a consumer from buying a homeopathic product made under unsanitary or unregulated conditions.

3. <u>Check the quality of the ingredients in your homeopathic glandular formula.</u> It is best to use a quality homeopathic formula which utilizes other homeopathic ingredients which have been proven to support the entire endocrine system. Be sure the glandulars used are from a company that attains them from range fed livestock free of herbicides and pesticides, synthetic fertilizers, or growth hormones. It is often best to get glandulars from New Zealand, because it is illegal in New Zealand to send dirty livestock to packing plants and animals are washed and inspected pre and post mortem. If there is a problem with the carcass of the animal or any of the origins, both are destroyed during this type of rigorous inspection. This is not the case in other areas of the world such as Great Britain, Europe, or Canada where animals have been exposed to BSE which is also known as Mad Cow Disease.

In my experience using homeopathic glandular blends, I have found that dosing with five to ten drops three to four times per day provides great results. Every bottle will; however, provide its own amounts and directions. Remember, using a homeopathic blend utilizing glandulars and other beneficial ingredients can support the entire endocrine system, making it more effective in rebalancing the body. Homeopathic medicine tends to be formulated to work best in blends.

4. <u>Understand the best way to use your low calorie ketogenic/glandular protocol for fat loss.</u> As described in Chapter 3, you want to be sure your overall calories are low enough to cause a state of deficit in the body, where it needs additional calories to survive. This will allow the hypothalamus, stimulated by the homeopathic glandulars, to stimulate the fat cells to release fat into the bloodstream to be used for fuel. It is essential that daily caloric intake is no higher than 500-800 calories to allow

for this process. As the other homeopathic glandulars work on balancing cortisol and estrogen with progesterone, this further facilitates the woman being able to achieve a ketogenic (fat-burning) state. The diet should be extremely low in fat to allow the body to use its own fat for fuel, and should be an approximate ratio of fifty percent low glycemic carbohydrates and fifty percent lean protein. Normally ketogenic diets are high in fat, because dietary fat is not going to cause fat storage in anyone (carbohydrates do that), but in this case, the fat needs to be low to allow the body to go in and take the fat stores to allow for efficient fat-burning.

2. I found that if we allowed clients to go over four weeks on this type of protocol, their weight loss can slow, which can be discouraging and can cause deviance. I recommend doing four- weeks-on, one-week-off before doing another round of four weeks of the low calorie ketogenic/glandular protocol. In the week off, I recommend eating higher-fat and protein foods with some limited low glycemic fruit, plenty of vegetables, but zero starch and sugar. These foods are similar to any low carbohydrate diet, but during these weeks "off" the low calorie ketogenic/glandular protocol, there are no calorie restrictions. This four-weeks-on, one-week-off, before starting another round of the low calorie ketogenic/glandular protocol for more weight loss is extremely effective, and yields a consistent twenty-pound per month loss for the average female client, and thirty-pound per month loss for men. This statement is also a little conservative, as some woman can lose ten to twenty-five percent more weight than that. Also note that it is essential to keep on track by making sure you do a "maintenance" phase for a full twenty-one days, and that you do it correctly. It is easy to lose weight quickly and then feel it is unnecessary to participate in this essential phase. This phase will "dry the concrete" on the weight lost during the weight-loss phase. If done incorrectly, the weight can easily come back on, as stated clearly by Dr. Simeons in his protocol using hCG. We mimic our maintenance phase for three weeks (about twenty one days) after Dr. Simeons

protocol and then slowly add in a few starches at a time after the three weeks.

5. <u>Consider liver support while losing weight on your low calorie ketogenic/glandular protocol.</u> The liver must work hard to break down all of the toxins that are released from your fat, which will be more rapid than normal on this type of protocol. I have gathered from all I have seen and read that weight loss in the United States can be a bit slower on average than in Europe or other less developed counties on a similar protocol (like hCG), due to the fact that our fat stores contain more toxins than the fat stores of Europeans. Weight loss can be slowed based on an individual's liver capacity. I suggest using an herbal supplemental liver support to aid in phase I and phase II detoxification of the liver. Herbs such as milk thistle, burdock, dandelion or even food concentrates like lemon juice, artichoke leaf extract, beet leaf or parsley leaf will all aid in this process. Food concentrates are more easily and safely taken than herbs because herbs can sometimes interfere with medications. The herbs mentioned are not as likely to cause interactions if they are not overdosed, but please remember to let your doctor know that you are taking them in conjunction with your medication. If you are on medications and are not working under a practitioner's supervision, then be sure to stick more closely with the food concentrates mentioned. While on the low calorie ketogenic/glandular protocol, these can be taken in concentrated supplements as well as consumed through herbal teas.

We use a professional strength, high quality liver support product called HepraCell in our Becoming Balanced...Hormonal Metabolic Correction Program. Be sure to read over the herbal ingredients to see if they may interact with your medications. We have used this product for several years with clients on every common medication and have seen no adverse affects. These herbs are not administered in high dosages and it would be rare for them to cause any medical interactions, but it is always best to check with your doctor.

There is another simple thing that you can do to assist the liver so that it is better able to process toxins. Deep relaxation therapy such as yoga, meditation, or "sound-wave" therapy—which will be mentioned later in this chapter—can serve to relax and "open up" the liver to allow for more efficient processing of toxins for faster weight loss.

6. Consider digestive imbalances while on your low calorie ketogenic/ glandular protocol. A simple free Candida yeast saliva test, also found on our website, can be taken to see if you have excess Candida yeast in your system. We all need a small amount of intestinal yeast, but the key is balance. When your good bacteria are killed off from coffee, stress, certain medications, or the BCP (see more in Chapter 5), then this gap allows for naturally occurring yeast to overgrow and cause problems. If you do not rid your body of excess Candida yeast by building up friendly digestive bacteria, you may gain some weight back easily after the thirty days on the low calorie ketogenic/glandular protocol is complete. When you have excess yeast in the body, it causes you to have strong cravings - and when you reintroduce starches, excess bloating and eventual weight gain can occur. Many people deal with daily yeast-related symptoms, but do not notice them until they do this simple test. A professional strength probiotic will help to resolve this issue by implanting good bacteria into the intestinal wall and increasing gut flora. A supplement with five-billion to twenty-billion in strength, in a one to four pills per day regimen, is beneficial to take when on your homeopathic glandular protocol. This is an optimal time to do so, since the low calorie ketogenic/glandular protocol is very low sugar and lends itself well to some natural die-off of yeast. A "human strain" friendly bacteria blend is more effective than most store-bought "plant strain" or "animal strain" products, which are not as natural to the body. You can test your Candida yeast levels after completing the low calorie ketogenic/glandular protocol, to see your improvement in friendly bacteria shown by a decrease in your Candida levels. If you still fail the saliva

test, continue on the therapeutic dose as stated above until your test is negative for Candida. Afterward, a simple dose of two to three probiotic pills per week (of capsules containing five to ten billion cells) can be used as a maintenance dosage. It is important to note that good levels of friendly bacteria will aid in most digestive conditions. We use a professional, high quality probiotic product called Flora-3 as part of our Becoming Balanced...Hormonal Metabolic Correction Program. You will receive the simple Candida saliva test along with the program.

7. Learn your food sensitivities as you finish your low calorie ketogenic/glandular protocol, and begin to add foods back into your diet. Many people have sensitivities to certain foods, most commonly dairy and wheat products. A food sensitivity is not a food allergy, which can cause an immediate and strong (possibly lethal) reaction in the body. Sensitivities are more subtle and are considered sub-clinical since they are not noticed by medical food testing for allergies. Knowing your food sensitivities is essential because the digestive disturbances resulting from them can eventually lead to weight gain after completing your low calorie ketogenic/glandular protocol. As you add back in dairy and wheat flour foods, it is a great time to make note of any unpleasant affects resulting from the consumption of these foods. A simple test we teach in my center is called The Coca Pulse Test by Dr. Arthur Coca. This test is based upon the principle that stress caused by intolerant foods will accelerate your pulse rate, therefore increases in the pulse rate after ingesting particular foods can identify sensitivity to those foods.

This simple, free test can be done in a few minutes after of taking your pulse in the morning, and then again later in the day for a few days to note your average pulse, and how much it can vary through the day. After this average is attained, you can take your pulse before and after a food you suspect being "sensitive" to, in order to note if it goes up by ten or more beats/minute. You may try it after a food depending on how it makes you feel when you first introduce it into your diet. This can be part of the process to tell if it "agrees" with you. You may have consumed some possibly "sensitive" foods your entire life, but since most people are used to not feeling their best, and often mix many foods in a meal, this sensitivity may have never been realized. Take advantage of this time of having a "clean slate" after the simple diet you were on for four or eight weeks, to notice how you feel. If you feel excessively thirsty, bloated, and sleepy, or have a headache or stomach ache, these are all clues that this is not a good food for you to continue eating. Food is fuel, and you should not feel uncomfortable if it is the right fuel for your body. In my BeBalanced center, we have always found that the book Eat Right 4 Your Type (see resources) is a great reference to start with, in order to see what foods to avoid for your particular blood type. However, always go by how you feel and let your intuition supersede what any book says if there seems to be a conflict.

8. Keep your hormones balanced after your low calorie ketogenic/ glandular protocol to anchor your success. In Chapter 3 it was explained how glandulars can aid in balancing your hormones (PMS/menopause symptoms reduced), and facilitate rapid fat loss when paired with the correct diet protocol. It is important to note that you will most likely not be able to sustain your new goal weight or your symptom management if your hormones become imbalanced again due to stress. Below are suggestions on how to prevent this:

a. Educate yourself on how the balance of estrogen and progesterone is key to maintaining your weight after the low calorie ketogenic/ glandular protocol (see Chapter 1).

b. Understand that the homeopathic glandular blends coupled with the ketogenic state will naturally raise progesterone levels and calm the adrenal gland, which needs to produce the stress hormone cortisol. This rebalancing causes the cessation of almost all symptoms of PMS and menopause. Following your weight loss; however, when the homeopathic glandular is discontinued and the full state of ketosis will stop, progesterone levels will fall again due to adrenal stress taking over. This results in the conversion of your progesterone into cortisol. In turn, this will cause "estrogen dominance" again, which will make weight gain likely, as well as allow for the return of many of your symptoms. When you do not feel well mentally and do not sleep well, you tend to make poor lifestyle choices, i.e. skipping your workout and eating junk food. Excessive exercise and severe calorie restriction to try to compensate for the weight gain can exacerbate your hormonal imbalance, and will tend to lead to additional weight gain. It is essential to keep the newly attained hormonal balance you achieved with the low calorie ketogenic/glandular protocol in order to "protect your investment." The best way to do this, after finishing the low calorie ketogenic/glandular protocol, is to use some sort of progesterone therapy while also addressing your adrenal fatigue/exhaustion, as mentioned in Solution #1

#1. This vital step will keep your PMS and menopausal symptoms at bay, so you feel your best and make healthy lifestyle decisions. The other main benefit of adding Solution #1

#1. After you have lost weight, due to ketosis achieved with the homeopathic glandular, is to allow you to maintain your new weight due to no longer being "estrogen dominant," which is often associated with weight gain in many women.

Precautions for Solution #2

A minor precaution to mention with the use of a low fat, low calorie ketogenic diet protocol is that sometimes people with pre-existing gall stones can have this issue worsen, and come to a head during the time. This is simply due to the fact that the diet protocol is very low in fat, and fat is needed for bile to flow easily from the gallbladder. Though this is very rare, it is worth mentioning, although I have not experienced any issues with this in my clients. This is most likely due to the fact that we only allow thirty days (one round) on the low calorie ketogenic/glandular protocol, and then a week is taken off (between rounds), where we encourage higher fat foods and Omega oils three, six and nine.

Another precaution with this low calorie ketogenic/glandular protocol is to watch certain medications, as the dosage may need to be lowered (with your doctor's supervision) to ensure that you are not over-medicated. This can happen sometimes as early as your first or second week on the protocol. If you are not paying attention to this, you could end up feeling tired or faint. The medications to really monitor are the ones that treat blood sugar and blood pressure, as your blood sugar and blood pressure tend to stabilize quickly with the healthy foods and achievement of hormonal balance. Cholesterol will be lowered as well, but this is not as pertinent to monitor. Your levels can be checked by your doctor at your next cholesterol screening. Also, the thyroid stabilizes fairly quickly, and if you are on a synthetic thyroid medication, like Synthroid, you tend to feel good, calm, and you sleep better initially. However, as your thyroid stabilizes, you will tend to need less medication, especially if you do more than one thirty day round on the low calorie ketogenic/glandular protocol. If you do not get retested and lower your medication with your doctor, you will probably feel jittery, over-stimulated, and not be able to sleep. This is serious, since being overmedicated on thyroid medications can be harmful, and can possibly create a dangerous condition called a "thyroid storm."

These are the predominant medication modifications that we see with our clients. You can feel free to go off of depression and anxiety medications as you feel better (read more in Chapter 6). Weaning off of these medications can be done with your doctor's assistance. There is always the chance that as you get healthier, these medications will make you feel worse if not eliminated. Most of my female clients report to me that they no longer need these strong psychotropic drugs after their hormones are balanced, and that they also feel "more alive" and "think more clearly" without them.

In conclusion, let it be emphasized that a low calorie ketogenic/glandular protocol can work even for the most stubborn weight issues, and is an excellent solution for women over forty who struggle with these hormonal weight issues. It will not only balance estrogen and progesterone, but it will also reset the whole metabolism. The homeopathic glandular blend can positively affect the hypothalamus and the pituitary gland, in addition to the thyroid and sex glands. Our version of this program is called Becoming Balanced and can be found at your local BeBalanced center. See locations at www. bebalancedcenters.com. The Becoming Balanced program comes complete with our Metabolic Correction Blend utilizing glandulars and other support, an herbal liver aid, a professional strength probiotic, and a "sound- wave" therapy CD accompanied by an eye pillow and aromatherapy. You will also receive the paperwork and the in person or phone appointments to guide you through the process. We also offer support for questions on medications or special issues. Our natural hormone balancing creams, ProPlus and Soothe Stress, can also be purchased at your local BeBalanced center (see website for locations) in order to begin to anchor your results as you complete the low calorie ketogenic/glandular protocol and enter into the twenty one days of maintenance.

Section 3

Solution #3 The use of HGH for Aging due to the Hormone Shift . . . relieving symptoms related to premature aging

After reading Chapter 7, The Hormone Shift & Aging, you can see that it is not vanity, but rather a true desire to maintain vitality that may motivate you to use HGH along with a full health protocol. Cost no longer has to be an issue with a homeopathic form of HGH and there are no documented side effects.

Know what you are buying

The only way to achieve the benefits mentioned in Chapter 7 is to use real injectable HGH, which needs a doctor's prescription and is about one thousand dollars per month, or use a true homeopathic form of HGH. Some companies say "homeopathic-like" and distribute it in pill or sublingual form. This is a dead giveaway that it is not real HGH. The molecules of HGH are too large to be absorbed under the tongue or to go through the normal digestive process. Sublingual forms of HGH are only effective in a homeopathic form.

Benefits of Homeopathic HGH over regular HGH:

1) Homeopathic HGH is safe. There are no documented side effects or drug interactions; this is true with almost all homeopathic formulas.

2) Homeopathic HGH is easy to use. Simply spray or drop under the tongue daily; no injections necessary.

3) Homeopathic HGH is less expensive than the real HGH as this can run up to a thousand dollars per month.

4) Homeopathic HGH uses low doses with high frequency, proven by studies to work as the best dosing for HGH.

5) Homeopathic HGH gently encourages the pituitary gland to release and supplement the body with natural HGH, which decreases with time. This means it aids the body in balance or homeostasis.

What to look for in an HGH product

1) Be sure it is a true homeopathic blend as only this or an injectable form will provide results. A real homeopathic formula will include the potencies on the label, as 3x, 30x, or 2C, 3C etc.

2) Be sure it is hand succussed (shaken) for optimal results, which is preferred over machine succussed formulas as this is more in line with the core principles of homeopathy.

3) It is advisable that it comes from an FDA-approved lab; the FDA has no official opinion on the efficacy of homeopathic medicine other than concern with safety, purity, ingredients, and claims.

The best way to take Homeopathic HGH

Take one to two sprays or three to five drops of homeopathic HGH in the morning upon rising, three to five drops between 3:00-6:00 PM and three to five drops in the evening upon retiring. This should be done for the first month. A one ounce bottle will last for one month if carefully measured out on a spoon. After thirty days, the HGH will have re-trained your system and is then only needed twice a day. A helpful hint is to keep the bottle on your nightstand and take the two doses, stated above, in the morning and upon retiring. At this rate, a one ounce bottle will last six weeks.

Benefits of our Homeopathic HGH: Essence of Youth

I have used homeopathic HGH for a number of years and have incorporated it into my center for my clients after they lose weight on our low calorie ketogenic/glandular protocol and after they have successfully stabilized their sex hormones. It works best when sex hormones are balanced and at optimal levels.

We named our formula Essence of Youth and it can be ordered directly from the Lancaster, Pa. BeBalanced Center.

- Our *Essence of Youth* is hand succussed (shaken) in potencies as high as 3x and 30x. You do not want machinery to shake the blend as EMF (electromagnetic field) "vibrations" of the machinery can affect the pure "vibrations" of the homeopathic solution.

- Our *Essence of Youth* comes from a laboratory that is FDA-approved for making homeopathic remedies.

- Our *Essence of Youth* has other homeopathic properties which aid the hypothalamus, thyroid and the pituitary gland. Homeopathic formulas work well when blended because they produce better overall results.

- Our homeopathic blend is one of the most inexpensive homeopathic HGH products available on the Internet. We buy in bulk quantities and can pass savings on to the client.

The Protocol for taking HGH

I recommend following a larger protocol if using homeopathic HGH for enhanced effects (stated below) because it allows you to take a more active role in your health. I have clients that use our Essence of Youth anywhere along their path to balancing hormones and weight, but below I outline when it is best to add it to your regimen if you so desire.

1. Use homeopathic HGH after you lose weight with Solution #2 and have stabilized your sex hormones with a form of progesterone therapy (as suggested in Solution #1). You may also add it into your regimen while on our low calorie ketogenic/ glandular protocol if you decide to do a second or third round because it can enhance the weight loss results for some people. I feel it is best not to use HGH with your first round of our low calorie ketogenic/glandular protocol so as to establish your average weight loss per month initially.

2. Use homeopathic HGH while balancing your sex hormones with Solution #1 (when no weight loss is needed). Using HGH along with your chosen form of progesterone therapy and adrenal support will further enhance its results. HGH always works best if sex hormones are at optimal levels, so always use Solution #1 for two to four weeks first before adding Solution #3 (HGH).

3. Go right into the HGH protocol I have outlined below with your choice of homeopathic HGH. This would be if you do not need to lose weight and already have your sex hormones balanced. It may also be used if you are already on some sort of hormone therapy to enhance effects with skin, muscle tone, sleep, etc.

The below protocol is one that I set in place at my center and can be used with any HGH method that you may choose. This protocol is based on all of the studies on HGH and is a holistic approach to better health.

-   Practice daily stress management. This means turning the mind off for twenty to thirty minutes while triggering deep, slow breathing and slowed brainwave patterns. This is getting out of the sympathetic nervous system, which is your "fight or flight" response, and into the anti-aging, immune building, energy giving para-sympathetic nervous system which rebalances the body. Read more on simple, effective ways to do this in Section 4.

- Practice daily movement to dispel stress while incorporating resistance training two to three times per week. Our bodies lose 1% of our muscle mass each year as we age if it is not tended to. Any type of resistance training done twice in a ten-day period is all that is needed to maintain muscle mass. This then leaves you free to do any daily movement that you actually enjoy along with some added stretching or yoga to maintain flexibility.

- Lower refined carbohydrates, in the forms of white sugar and white flour, to a minimum of one to two (if any) servings per day.

- Go to bed at a reasonable hour and aim for deep restorative sleep of at least eight hours each night. This deeper sleep will happen on HGH but you must provide the time or simply get in bed so it can happen.

Adding HGH to a foundation of healthy lifestyle choices and natural hormonal therapy can give "icing on the cake" results!

A Bit about Homeopathic Medicine

Before we get into the ways in which homeopathic remedies work, I want to mention that if you take a homeopathic formula like HGH, it is best to not eat or drink anything fifteen to twenty minutes before or after taking the drops. It is also best to avoid coffee close to the time at which you take a dosage because coffee is known to interfere with the vibrations of homeopathic substances. Also, avoid storing the bottle in extreme heat or by electrical appliances, such as microwaves. The chaotic frequencies emitted from certain appliances can throw off the vibrations of the remedy.

Next, I would like to briefly discuss the background of homeopathy and how it works. It may not necessarily be the easiest thing to comprehend, but ask yourself, "Do I fully comprehend how that little yellow pill works that I take to make my headache go away?" Just do your best to understand the concept behind homeopathic medicine similarly to how you try to comprehend the working mechanics of a prescription drug. Please keep in mind what we discussed; homeopathic formulas are far safer than prescription drugs.

Homeopathy is a type of alternative medicine that has been utilized in our country since the European settlers came to America. The basic principle of homeopathy is "let like be cured by like." Homeopathic formulas work by influencing the body with vibrations, which is more in line with influencing the energy of the body. You can relate this to the ancient practice of acupuncture. This type of science is more directly related to the physics of the body and its energy vibrations, rather than solely the biochemistry of the cell. Homeopathy looks beyond the microscopic parts of the cell and works at the level of the protons, neutrons and electrons. Standard allopathic medicine, which is popular in America, is more prone to influence the chemistry and biology of the body. Its purpose is to see how the cells react to change with certain foods, herbs or drugs. In my opinion, homeopathic formulas are safer than drugs, but they are also just as, if not more, effective than the original drug substances used to make many of them (example, HGH). This is because any substance (even a prescription drug) put into a homeopathic form, will not tax the liver and stress the body with all of the additional side effects.

While most prescription drugs treat the symptoms of a disease, homeopathy is intended to treat the root of a problem, which is often connected to the energy of the body. Homeopathy looks to find the cause of the symptoms that are often due to subtle imbalances in the system. These imbalances, as you have learned, are sometimes hormonal. Homeopathy promotes healing and strength in the body and helps to restore balance.

In homeopathy, a substance, such as a drug, steroid, herb, or vitamin, is diluted down several times in distilled water, combined with alcohol to stabilize it, and is usually noted in dilutions of 1x, 2x, 3x . . . 100x. The more diluted the substance, the "weaker" it becomes; therefore, the fewer side effects it would have versus its original state. Surprisingly however, the "vibration" is raised and it has a more powerful effect on the body. This is because the substance becomes purer, and therefore its original impurities are negligible. Dilutions can even go as far as eliminating all of the molecules from the original substance. However, it still influences the body just the same. If you wish to understand homeopathic medicine on a deeper level then please refer to Appendix G for a continuation of this discussion.

Section 4

A Solution to Stress that caused the Hormone Shift . . .
making all of the solutions work better!

My hope is that you now have a better grasp on how the combination of physical, mental and emotional stress equals our total "stress load." This overall stress load is what our adrenal gland must endure and is the key factor in causing all sex and stress hormone imbalances. In this section I plan to explain what you can actively do to compensate for the total stress load in your life so it has less of an impact on your hormonal balance. Unfortunately, the American lifestyle makes these lifestyle adjustments not only beneficial but fully necessary for optimal hormonal balance.

Relaxation Therapy for Ultimate Hormone Balance

Our inactive modern culture is unlike that of our ancestors. The body instinctually wants to move, so living in today's society we must figure out a way to compensate for our desk jobs. Oddly, but all too commonly, Americans drive to the gym so that they may participate in thirty-minutes of aerobics or weight lifting in order to help offset all of those hours of sitting. This must seem so strange to older generations who were just naturally more active. However, the result of the thirty-minutes of exercise allows us to feel better, burn calories, lower blood pressure, and helps us to be healthier in so many ways.

The same is true for stress. Our minds were intended to be free of too much stimulation, worry, fear or stress; but even in our happiest times, we are over-stimulated mentally. We initiate what is known as the "stress response." It is the daily sympathetic nervous system's response of "fight- or-flight." However, because we do not literally have to run away from a lion or a bear, we do not get the overall benefits of the exercise, meaning we do not burn off the excess stress hormone (cortisol) produced. Instead, the adrenal gland becomes exhausted and our sex hormones become imbalanced. The parasympathetic nervous system is where the body digests, heals and regenerates, and where our immune system can build. This is where we should be functioning everyday but most often we are not. In order for us to function better in this parasympathetic mode, which aids our mood and our overall healing, we must incorporate regular relaxation therapy.

Consider taking action to reduce your mental and emotional stress so that you can eliminate bad habits such as overeating and inactivity. Quite often, if you are anxious, depressed, or in a bad mood, you will reach for a sugary, starchy treat and head for the couch rather than the gym.

Dr. Herbert Benson, an associate professor of medicine at the Harvard Medical School, studied stress and its many links to disease; both physical and mental. He determined that if we could evoke what is called a "relaxation response" every day, it will have long-term and wide-spread positive ramifications for the body and mind. He essentially is the pioneer for this theory and is the author of a book titled The Relaxation Response. He goes on to say that if we can offset the stress response, it will vastly improve our health and assist in issues such as weight loss. The "relaxation response" is defined by the very relaxed brainwave patterns that occur. These slowed brainwave patterns are even slower than when napping or sleeping at night. They start with the high activity of Gamma/ Beta waves (13-40 Hz) during a stressful day and then move to the slightly relaxed Alpha waves (8-12 Hz), then progress to Theta waves (4-7 Hz) as we go to sleep, and lastly the slowest waves called Delta (1-3 Hz) where regeneration can be achieved. Delta brainwave patterns are difficult to achieve even during sleep in our stress-filled modern society, but have been documented during times of meditation, yoga practice, massage, and deep prayer. Specific tools that aid us in deep relaxation tend to be needed to reach these brainwave patterns in an awakened state. Certain types of special music therapy can be combined with meditation (a release of thoughts), or guided imagery (a focus on positive words/images which curtails negative stressful thinking). This combination can guide you to positive behavioral changes. I love how I feel when I practice relaxation therapy and attain these Delta brainwave patterns. My first introduction to this type of relaxation therapy was through the work of Kelly Howell and the company, Brain Sync. This type of music is a form of "sound-wave" therapy, called brainwave synchronization music, and was first discovered by biophysicist Gerald Oster of the Mount Sinai Hospital in New York City. Kelly Howell further pioneered this field by creating programs for scientists and medical professionals such as Harvard-trained neurosurgeon, Norman Shealy. His programs were often recommended to various cancer treatment hospitals such as Memorial Sloan-Kettering. EEG studies conducted at Harvard Body-Mind Medical School and UCLA concluded that brainwave synchronization music shift s brainwave patterns. I use this type of music therapy (or "sound-wave" therapy) for an in-house relaxation therapy program described below.

To further evoke the "relaxation response," it is best to start by locating the causes of stress in your life (see Chapter 1), and then come up with a plan to lower these factors—for example: more sleep, physical therapy, chiropractic care, or even less processed foods. The other things that cause you stress such as your marriage, children, job, and finances may be a bit more difficult to change but these should be assessed as well in order to implement creative ways to lower your existing stress. A better attitude or slight adjustment in attitude could also be a simple solution. This "life assessment" may take some thought and time but it will aid in better balancing your hormones. This will also translate to the overall quality of your life, slow the aging process and prevent certain diseases. See the "Lighten Up Emotionally Exercise" in Appendix A.

Benefits of Relaxing and Reaching Delta Brainwaves

* Decreases overall stress; physical, mental and emotional

* Decreases stress on the liver, allowing it to work more efficiently at breaking down fat and detoxifying the body for optimal weight los

* Decreases binge and stress eating, as well as aids in healthy lifestyle choices

* Improves sleeping patterns

* Increases energy, which is necessary for exercise

* Improves memory and concentration

* Balances sex hormones (estrogen & progesterone) to aid in proper thyroid function, PMS, fertility problems, fluid and fat loss

* Balances blood sugar (insulin levels) to reduce cravings and increase your fat burning potential

* Decreases blood pressure and stress on the heart muscle

* Decreases all stress-related digestive problems (like IBS)

* Decreases stress hormones (cortisol), increasing immunity while decreasing abdominal fat deposits

* Provides an "emotional release" for pent-up emotions that can cause poor health or bad moods

* Promotes the release of "feel-good" chemicals in the brain

In my center, we use a program I developed over twelve years ago called, *Conditioned Response*, that utilizes "sound-wave" therapy, guided visualization and aromatherapy (includes an eye pillow). My work on this program was published in the international magazine called Aromatherapy and Wellbeing, May/June 2002. We use this program in our Becoming Balanced...Hormonal Metabolic Correction Program for enhanced weight loss as I feel relaxation therapy is essential in our modern world and key to weight loss efforts.

The sound waves patterns under the music on the *Conditioned Response* relaxation program are meant to deeply relax the mind to reach slow Delta waves which will then transfer to a deeply relaxed body. This nourishes all systems to allow for the healing needed in our stressful lives. The idea behind this theory uses the Pavlovian model of simple "classical conditioning." After a few weeks of cultivating a relaxed state every day while inhaling the essential oils, a *Conditioned Response* will form between the scent and the feeling of peace/ euphoria. This response is a great form of "aroma" therapy and can monumentally help in breaking people out of the "fight or flight" mode of the sympathetic nervous system that we function in all too often. Stopping a few times in your stress-filled day to relax and do some deep breathing will be further enhanced when inhaling these essential oils.

The idea of combining scent with relaxation stems from the work of renowned neurologist, Dr. Allen Hirsh, who runs the *Smell and Taste Treatment and Research Foundation* in Chicago, Illinois. His (1998) book called *Scentsational Weight Loss* proved with a study of over 3,000 participants that scent alone (without exercise, diet or relaxation) could induce a weight loss of an average of five to six pounds per month when participants were asked to smell a synthetic fragrance throughout the day before eating or when cravings persisted. It was as simple as that, and the resultant decrease in eating caused the weight loss. Dr. Hirsh, a specialist in scent and smell, goes on to explain the relationship between scent and satiety in his book. He was even kind enough to meet with me for lunch, years ago in Chicago, to discuss the idea of my program of combining scent with relaxation in order to form a *Conditioned Response* while using pure aromatherapy (as opposed to synthetic scents). Scent alone can increase satiety (and decrease cravings), but a pure aromatic blend will tend to work even better due to the amazing properties of essential oils with molecules that are so small they can easily pass into the limbic (emotional) center of the brain. Most studies on using essential oils for "aroma" therapy have been performed in Europe where it is literally considered a valid form of therapy (see references for books on aromatherapy and the psyche). My theory was that if this scent were then attached to a memory of relaxation (with a strong physiological response) there should be a lasting calming impact when purposely inhaled during a stressful day. This "relaxation response" would also, of course, increase satiety (decrease appetite) if the blend is dabbed under the nose. Any strong scent will have a similar effect but this oil blend will take this effect to the next level due to the calm feeling now associated with it after using it in the full program.

I overlaid Track One of the relaxation program with verbiage. This allows for visualization work that relates to a "new slimmer body" so it further adds positive benefits. We accept positive suggestions better in a relaxed state. Any of the following can be used to relax and evoke behavior/thought changes; guided imagery, visualization work, or self-hypnosis (specifically implanting ideas into your mind for use in specific behavior modification). All three of these work with the subconscious mind in a relaxed state by making gentle suggestions for behavioral changes that are meant to influence you after the session is complete throughout your day. I found that when using music/sound therapy, overlaid with some guided imagery, you tend to occupy the right side of the brain (emotionally-based) with the music and the left side of the brain (logically-based) with the words.

Years ago when I had shared this theory with a local neurobehavioral psychologist, Robert Stein Ph.D., he emphasized that scent would be a legitimate "anchor" or post-hypnotic cue to be used after a session of listening to the *Conditioned Response* program which was in fact a form of self hypnosis. The scent would help remind the person of relaxation, satiety, and contentment (emphasized in the wording on the relaxation program) serving as a post-hypnotic cue or suggestion outside the trans-like state. In this case, I used an aromatic scent as a strong cue tied to a relaxed, satiated, and content feeling.

Post-hypnotic cues are important and are a powerful extension of any relaxation therapy. These cues will allow you to change or improve your behavior and responses anytime throughout your day. One reason these post-hypnotic cues work so well is because your unconscious mind uses memories to provoke an action or a response that you would have implanted while in a relaxed state (also called self-hypnosis). This has been demonstrated countless times in clinical research.

I tested this theory of guided imagery and sound-wave therapy combined with essential oils with many of my clients and found this simple theory to be extremely effective. I do admit that it was (and still is) hard to get a woman to lie down and relax for twenty to thirty minutes in her busy day! Hopefully after reading the proven benefits of relaxation therapy and better understanding the havoc that stress can cause on our hormones, this may be more readily done.

The essential oil blend that is part of the *Conditioned Response* program can be used at any time to bring you back into the relaxed trance-like state. To further enhance the *"relaxation response"* brought on by breathing in the scent is the fact that the oils chosen for the program are physiologically sedating (relaxing to the central nervous system) and psychologically uplifting to the mood (fighting depression anxiety). Used throughout your stressful day, the essential oil blend will improve mood as well as decrease appetite.

I tested this specific oil blend with a local neurologist who offered his time and equipment (EEG machine). It was amazing to see on the printout that inhaling the pure essential oil blend alone (even without the *Conditioned Response* effect) influenced a state of relaxation in the brain.

The essential oil blend for the *Conditioned Response* program was originally formulated by Rose Linkens of Restoration Spa, Lancaster, PA. She is an internationally board-certified CIDESCO* diplomat and the first United States esthetician to achieve CIDESCO diploma in aromatherapy. As a result, she has presented around the world the benefits of aromatherapy.

CIDESCO stands for Comite International d'Esthetique et de Cosmetologie in French and International Committee for Esthetics and Cosmetology in English. The CIDESCO diploma is one of the world's most prestigious in the field of aesthetics and beauty therapy.

Only pure essential oils are used in the *Conditioned Response* program and each contain hundreds of beneficial chemical constituents. It is best to keep pure essential oil blends in dark bottles to protect their beneficial properties. Below are some of the main oils; blended in a specific ratio:

Benzoin (comfort)
Sandalwood (relaxing, sedative)
Frankincense (balancing)
Patchouli (uplifting)
Elemi (refreshing)

This program can be implemented as part of your daily routine, even well past the point that your weight loss goals have been attained. I encourage you to research other relaxation tracks on-line in order to expand your library of options to be used for your daily quiet time (see resources). The Conditioned Response program is included in our Becoming Balancing... Hormonal Metabolic Correction program through your local BeBalanced Center.

Hopefully, you feel as if there is now hope to look and feel the way that you did prior to your hormone Shift . It is possible for women to become more confident and independent with age. If you can combine your wisdom and your innate intuition with feeling and looking more youthful, you can have it all. You must believe it and work towards this change with these simple steps. Soon your mental mindset towards aging will "Shift", as your hormones "Shift back", and you will truly come to embrace the best years of your life!

Imagine . . .

What new outfit would you buy for your slimmer body?

How would you treat your husband when in that "better mood?"

How would your husband appreciate your increased libido?

What new passion would you delve into?

What dream would you make come true with your new outlook on life?

This gift of health and hormone balance would simply be the springboard for you to jump into the refreshing pool of life's unending possibilities! I am convinced that if you can feel as good as you were meant to feel, at that height, at that pinnacle, you would get a different view on how your life could be. But only you can do this for yourself. My goal in writing this book is to help remove any physical or mental barriers that were "hormonally-based" so that you can reach new heights of self-love and self-awareness—all leading to deeper intimacy in your relationships, improved parenting, increased creativity, better job productivity, and the ability to self-nurture.

If you are willing and dedicated to "becoming" all you were meant to be, it can all start with one step; it can all start in the next thirty days when you naturally work with your hormone rhythms!

There is a reason we use a butterfly in our company logo for the Becoming Balanced...Hormonal Metabolic Correction Program. It was well thought through . . .

Just when the caterpillar thought all hope was lost . . .
. . . it became a beautiful butterfly.
Let your inner butterfly fly free for the entire world to see!

CHAPTER 9

The Hormone Shift & Hair

The Use of Natural Hormone Balancing Methods to Reduce Hair Loss/Thinning....

What role do hormones and stress play in hair loss/thinning? What causes hair loss/thinning in women specifically when compared to hair loss in men?
What are the main physiological and psychological components of hair loss/thinning?
What are some natural ways to reverse hair loss/thinning?
Solution: Increase micro-circulation via a low sugar diet, topical therapies and stress management techniques while balancing sex and stress hormones.

I t seems like we've been talking about male pattern baldness and hair loss in men for years but only more recently have there been articles and information about hair loss for women. I believe this is because the subject was a bit taboo, combined with the fact that it was less common for women's hair to thin until they were perhaps in their eighties or nineties. Currently, along with the trend of women having worsening symptoms of mood, weight, and sleep around menopause, it seems like hair loss/ thinning is one of the top ten symptoms women are dealing with. The reason for this, I believe, is simply that hormone imbalances seem to be worse, and are reaching epidemic proportions. Increased stress, causing increased sugar/caffeine/ alcohol consumption, coupled with increased use of certain medications, are causing very dramatic hormonal swings and imbalances that are unique to our modern-day society. Blissful relaxation,- something to most Americans seems like a distant fantasy, could lower cortisol, rebalance sex and stress hormones, decrease cravings (with the resulting indulgences in sugar/

alcohol / caffeine), decrease the need for medication, and can relax scalp muscles and connective tissue to allow for increased microcirculation to the hair follicle. While moving to a dessert island to experience ultimate relaxation is probably not an option, we will explore in this chapter how to get similar hair rejuvenating results with supplementation, treatments, and some simple lifestyle changes.

To better help you understand therapy for hair loss, let us first establish a basis for hair loss itself. There are many causes of hair loss, but the main cause for both men and women - affecting about 50% of adult males and 25% of adult women, is directly related to changes in the hair's nutrition (based on circulation of blood to the follicle), hormone imbalances, and scalp hygiene.

Your scalp is composed of many layers that could negatively affect your hair growth if proper circulation is not maintained. The skin (epidermis, the dermis, and the subcutaneous layer) is only the surface. There are deeper layers of connective tissue, called fascia, and muscle with the scull as the foundation. Within all these layers there are blood vessels, nerves, and glands, and the hair (or keratin). All hair is supported by blood flow, which carries oxygen and nutrients to promote cellular activity and new growth. Proper circulation, as you will see, is key for hair growth and essential for healthy hair, because it will allow blood (oxygen) and nutrients to reach the papilla area (base of the hair follicle, fed by the blood via tiny capillaries). When there is a decrease in micro-circulation to the hair shaft, and fewer nutrients reach the papilla, the hair cells reproduce at a much slower rate. The result of this slower cellular activity produces thinner, poor quality hair.

Types of Hair Loss

There are different types of loss/thinning:

1. An overall thinning of hair where each individual hair strand gets thinner over time.

2. "Male pattern" balding; hair loss/thinning at temples and front of crown.

3. The dramatic loss/thinning of hair all over the head or in large patches due to a traumatic event. This can be associated with adrenal fatigue or failure.

What we will be discussing in this chapter can help with all of these types of hair loss/thinning over time. Each of these types of hair loss stated above, specifically number three, has a large stress component that originates with the adrenal gland, but all have a strong origin in a decrease in certain female hormones, an increase in stress hormones, and an imbalance in (androgenic) male hormones.

Current Hair Loss Solutions

Before we go on, let us quickly review some of the more popular current solutions out there for hair loss. The most popular of all is *Minoxidol*, which is a synthetic hair solution to be applied topically, which formerly was prescription only. The goal with *Minoxidol* is to increase vasodilatation of tiny blood vessels to aid in circulation to the hair follicle, and cause new growth in areas where follicles were possibly stunted. This solution is obviously temporary, and upon cessation, hair stops growing and will reverse to actually be worse than it was initially. This really surprised me when I learned this fact. It is one thing to say you need to use a product the rest of your life to maintain results, it is another thing to say you will revert back worse than where you were originally upon cessation of its use. I am not sure if that is a really smart marketing campaign to scare the customer into using it long-term, or just the truth that they are legally obligated to disclose. Besides this fun fact, there are some other side effects such as dry, flaky, itchy scalp (contact dermatitis), burning, stinging, or redness of the scalp, hypertrichosis (unwanted facial hair growth), increased hair loss (initially, but this can last for 2-3 months and is called "shedding"). If the solution is systemically absorbed, which is supposed to be rare, other symptoms can occurs such as dizziness, irregular heartbeat, fainting, light headedness, chest pain tiredness, difficulty breathing, neuritis (numbness or tingling of hands, feet, or face), sexual dysfunction or decreased libido, and visual disturbances such as blurred vision or decreased visual acuity... so perhaps you feel better because you can no longer see how much your hair is thinning! Another effect can be possible fluid retention which can cause headaches, weight gain, cardiac problems, and possibly high blood pressure for some people. Lastly, we are unsure of long-term safety of this product. Originally *Minoxidol* was for men, and then later they came out with a version for women that was a 2% solution as compared to the original 5% solution for men. I feel the jury is still out on this as a good therapy for women's hair loss/thinning, as many women report they have so much initial "shedding" or side effects that they quit using it in a few months, while others seem happy with the results.

The other popular way to get back your hair is usually advertised more for men who are completely bald in the front or on the top of their head. It is the surgical procedure using what is called "hair plugs." This is where live hair is transferred into areas where there is follicle death and no chance of re-growth. Obviously this can be very time-consuming, as well as painful and expensive. The results do seem very satisfactory for some men though.

Neither of these above two solutions, *Minoxidol* or hair plugs, gets to the bottom of the hormonal imbalance that is causing the hair loss/thinning. Of course using either of these solutions might give temporary results but there are no other health benefits like improved mood, sleep, and overall health such as when you use a more holistic approach that I like to take, which gets to the root of the problem.

Hair Rejuvenation Solution

The approach I like to take to aid in rejuvenating the hair and reversing the thinning and loss is multidimensional. Not only will results be faster, but the overall affect on a woman's health will be more profound. The core issue with hair loss is daily physiological as well as psychological stress. Daily, chronic stress causes many issues we need to address for proper hair growth:

- Hormones imbalances - High cortisol and imbalanced sex hormones, which can damage the hair follicle and alter growth phases, need to be balanced with supplements and simple lifestyle changes.

- Tight neck/scalp muscles- This results in restricted connective tissue (fascia) which decreases circulation to the hair follicle that needs to be loosened/relaxed via professional or personal techniques or therapies.

- Poor nutritional choices- Increased sugar consumption (decreases circulation over time)and less protein (needed for hair growth), as well as increased caffeine (depletes B vitamins needed for hair growth)and increased alcohol (increases hormone imbalances), all need to be addressed and replaced by foods that aid hair growth.

The approach of balancing hormones as a basis will lay the best foundation. This can be done by lifestyle changes (practicing some daily stress management) to facilitate hormone balancing, along with supplementation (to aid adrenal gland which handles the body's stress hormones) for faster hormonal balance. Additionally, any way you can increase micro- circulation will be helpful such as manual massage to loosen scalp muscles/ fascia or laser use. It is also essential to add in proper nutrition, so that the blood going to the follicles now brings nutrients needed for proper hair growth. The finishing touch that also makes logical sense is proper scalp hygiene, to keep follicles unblocked for stronger, thicker hair.

Key to this whole process of lowering stress is the ability to relax the mind, and let go of the worry about your hair loss. Hopefully this can be done as you now understand what causes it and what you can do to reverse it. Stress can be defined by lack of control, this process of working to get your hair healthy again gives you control, and something to focus on. This alone should help your cortisol go down due to less stressful thoughts about this problem. Relaxing your mind will relax muscles and increase circulation to the follicles. So as you read on, just glean from this chapter what you feel will work best for you, and begin to implement the healthy changes in your life.

Hormones & Hair Loss for Women

I will use a simple breakdown in bullet points that builds on what we discussed in Chapter 1. It is essential that you have that basic hormone education under your belt first.

- Increased simple sugar in the diet and well as alcohol and the overuse of caffeine increases the body's physiological stress and the stress hormone (cortisol), which then causes "insulin-resistance" ("insulin resistance" is explained more in Chapter 3 on weight loss).

- Increased daily psychological stress (job, family, finances, etc.) also increases cortisol, and also causes "insulin-resistance."

- "Insulin-resistance" increases the ability of testosterone in women to be converted to the androgen (male hormone) called DHT (dihydrotestosterone). DHT is a strong form of testosterone that in both men and women interacts with androgen receptors in scalp follicles, causing hair loss and decreased micro-circulation to the hair follicle.

- DHT specifically miniaturizes hair follicles by shortening the anagen (growth) phase and/or lengthening the telogen (resting) phase. This will almost always cause the hair follicles to slowly shrink and die. The long-term result is an increased number of short, thin, fine hairs barely visible above the scalp.

- Increased cortisol production, as stated in Chapter 1, also decreases female sex hormones needed to balance androgens like testosterone and DHT, making imbalances worse.

- Increased production of cortisol first will drain progesterone, but over time there is a "second-level depletion" causing estrogen levels to go down as well. This lowering of estrogen can occur after progesterone is low for a long time in a woman of any age, but naturally occurs around or after menopause. When this happens, you have the two major female hormones at a lower level, causing testosterone (then more DHT) to become more dominant, negatively impacting the hair follicle, and oftentimes resulting in hair loss/thinning.

The goal for optimal hair growth for women is to lower or stabilize cortisol levels via daily stress management techniques (coming up). Dietary changes need to be involved as well too (lower sugar, caffeine, and alcohol) as these will cause "insulin resistance," along with all the daily psychological stress women experience which raises cortisol and decreases circulation to the follicle. Additional tips coming up in this chapter will aid in this process as well.

Next is to add supplements which will raise progesterone levels, as this will keep a woman's testosterone from converting easily to DHT. Progesterone is the chief inhibitor of the enzyme 5-alpha reductase. Progesterone inhibits the body from converting testosterone to DHT by binding to 5 alpha reductase; 5-AR is the enzyme that converts testosterone into DHT.

Increasing progesterone, as mentioned many times in this book, is also needed to balance estrogen (pre-menopause), or to naturally raise estrogen if needed (after menopause). Progesterone really is the key to keeping estrogen in check, as well as testosterone. Raising progesterone is what we naturally do for women in my center for improvements in weight, mood, sleep, and overall female health, but is an essential foundation if you are trying to stimulate hair growth/ thickness.

For the purpose of balancing hormones to aid in hair loss, Chapter 8 talks about how to choose a natural progesterone cream to bring up progesterone levels and touches on our choice that we use in my center. This solution will aid in increasing progesterone (and estrogen indirectly) to balance male hormones in the body like testosterone, and keep it from converting to DHT.

However, in order to stabilize cortisol levels (beside typical stress management techniques and lowering sugar/ caffeine/ alcohol) some adrenal support is needed so that the body does not steal progesterone, and constantly convert that to cortisol. Adaptogenic herbs like ginseng or maca are good to balance and support the adrenal gland. Of course getting these ingredients into the body is always best sublingually (under the tongue) or via a trans-dermal (through the skin) cream to avoid weak or faulty digestion. This type of therapy will aid in balancing cortisol levels, so progesterone levels can rise properly, and prevent the conversion of testosterone to DHT.

Hormones & Hair Loss for Men

Men have a similar stress induced hormone imbalance causing hair loss/thinning. Below is a simple breakdown in bullet points that build on the basics of stress hormones that we discussed in Chapter 1. Keep in mind, men still need to keep the stress hormones low so as not to drain their vital sex hormones, but men also have a higher propensity for hair loss because they have more testosterone to begin with.

- Increased simple sugar in the diet as well as alcohol and the overuse of caffeine increases the body's physiological stress, and the stress hormone (cortisol) which then causes "insulin-resistance" ("insulin resistance" is explain more in Chapter 3 on weight loss).

- Increased daily psychological stress also increases cortisol and also causes "insulin-resistance."

- "Insulin-resistance" in men increases the ability of testosterone to be converted to the more potent form of testosterone called DHT.

- DHT interacts with androgen receptors in scalp follicles, and specifically miniaturizes hair follicles by shortening the anagen (growth) phase and/or lengthening the telogen (resting) phase. This will almost always cause the hair follicles to slowly shrink and die. The long-term result is an increased number of short, thin, fine hairs barely visible above the scalp.

- DHT will cause hair loss (male pattern baldness) and decreased micro-circulation to the hair follicle will cause men to grow more hair on their back and shoulders, and in their ears and nose as they age.

The goal for men is to lower stress with stress management techniques (similar as those to be explained for women) to stabilize cortisol which will allow testosterone to stabilize, so excess will not be converted to DHT and estrogens. Dietary changes need to be involved too (lower sugar caffeine and alcohol) as these will cause "insulin resistance" as well as daily stress. As previously stated for women, the additional tips in this chapter coming up will aid in this process as well.

It is also interesting to note that high levels of cortisol, due to stress that causes "insulin resistance," can also cause a man's testosterone to be more readily converted to estrogen which will can result in an enlarged prostate, increased moodiness, lowered libido, and sometimes gynecomastia (enlarged breasts). This scenario can also be linked to the rare cases of male breast cancer.

Just as in women, in order to stabilize cortisol levels (beside typical stress management techniques and lowering sugars, caffeine and alcohol), some adrenal support is needed so that the body does not steal testosterone and other hormone precursors (building blocks the body uses to make testosterone), and convert them into cortisol to fill this need for cortisol- based stress demands. Adaptogenic herbs like ginseng or maca are good to balance and support the adrenal gland. As stated for women, getting these ingredients into the body is always best sublingually (under the tongue) or via a trans-dermal (through the skin) cream to avoid weak or faulty digestion. This type of therapy will aid in balancing cortisol levels to aid in the "insulin resistance" program that converts testosterone to DHT, causing hair loss and male pattern baldness.

It seems like a simple solution to just take testosterone to aid in lowering levels that occur with age and stress, but most often this does not work since most men in our country are slightly to moderately "insulin resistant." In almost all cases when testosterone is taken directly, it will convert to estrogen, exacerbating any problems. If it were that simple, all men would simply just take testosterone when they reach a certain age. I do not work with men a lot, but in my limited experience, I have only seen straight testosterone benefit men in very rare cases, and these men were trim and healthy, having really taken care of themselves. Although I did not test them, I assume they were most likely not "insulin resistant." If a man wants to do some type of supplementation for aiding proper testosterone with age, and preventing its conversion to DHT, bedsides changing diet/ lifestyle habits as described in this chapter, I suggest hormone precursors. Precursors are "building blocks" from which the body can make cortisol or testosterone when needed, without any risks or overdoses. Examples of these would be DHEA and pregnenolone (often called a mother hormone), but these are most effective taken in trans- dermal cream form to bypass the digestive process. As I always recommend you want to be sure the topical hormone cream you are using is a true "trans-dermal," to be sure it gets into the bloodstream effectively and excretes in 18-24 hours. For more on this, see the section from our chemist in Chapter 8.

Since this book was written more for women than men, and I have not gone into too much depth on male hormones outside of this chapter on hair loss (more for comparison with women hair loss), please email us at info@bebalancedcenters.com for more information on our male support natural hormone cream.

Fascia and Muscle Release for Hair Growth

The scalp is formed by the movable soft tissue which should not be super tight so as not to cut off circulation to the hair follicles which is needed for growth. The basic layers of the scalp for the purpose of our discussion are:

- Skin - The skin is dense in sebaceous glands on the scalp, more than other places on the body.

- Superficial fascia - This is connective tissue that provides a passageway for nerves and blood vessels. Blood vessels are attached to this fibrous connective tissue. This is where I want to focus as this area get tighter and cut off blood supply to the follicles when we are under stress and underlying muscle gets tight.

- Occipitofrontalis muscle - This is the large muscle on the skull that extends to the back of the head from the front or brow line that can get tight when we are under stress.

- Subaponeurotic layer - This is another deeper layer of loose connective tissue.

- Pericranium - This layer helps attach the muscle to the bone

- Subpericranial connective tissue - Another layer of deeper connective tissue

- Skull bone

People know muscles get tight due to chronic stress but we forget about the fascia which is the thin but strong connective tissue that covers muscles and bones on the body including the skull. Healthy, normal fascia is flexible but it can get very tight and stiff over time and cutting off blood supply to the hair follicles. You should be able to move your scalp back and forth when you pull a bit on your hair. The more flexible the better. If you cannot move it at all and it feels really tight, this can be referred to as restricted fascia. Restricted fascia always leads to decreased circulation and inadequate oxygen supply, nutrients, water and hormones to the cells or in this case the hair follicles. When this occurs, along with sub-optimal food choices, lack of rest, and emotional stress, metabolic waste products can build up, contributing significantly to the aging of the cells or follicles. Myofascia release is a type of massage that release tension in the fascia and aids pain tremendously when standard massage, chiropractic and even physical therapy fails to stop chronic pain. This type of therapy can also be done on the scalp, I determined, to loosen the tight constrictions there to aid in increase blood supply which would then obviously aid hair growth and stimulation. Myofascia release goes beyond scalp massage in that techniques are applied using a compression movement moving towards the direction of restriction without any lubricant like oil or lotion. What this does is actually reduce tissue restriction allowing the body to use its own natural resources to improve the health of your hair so it grows more like it did when you were younger...faster, thicker, stronger!

I feel this is one very basic but key secret to reversing hair thinning that is overlooked when looking for solutions to this problem. I would go so far as to say if this is overlooked and a person does have restricted, tight fascia and muscles, the other topical treatments and diet changes will not yield optimal results due to this barrier of blood reaching the follicles.

Scalp Care for Hair Health

Another factor in hair thinning, or the cause of hair to be weaker, is overall scalp care. The scalp needs to be cleansed properly; using hair products that clog the delicate hair follicles should be avoided. Sebum buildup (sebaceous oil on the surface of the scalp) can collect in the hair follicle and harden, causing a sebum plug that can hinder hair growth. This will only compound pre-existing issues of the weak hairs, reducing hair growth further. Shampoos and even conditioners that contain extra moisturizers tend to clog hair follicles over time. In order to prevent this, it is best to use products labeled non-comedogenic, which means that they are formulated to prevent them from blocking hair follicles. Occasional, or at least weekly, use of a clarifying shampoo (shampoo that has no conditioning ingredients) will also help remove hair products like styling gels or mousse that tend to accumulate in the hair follicles and block them. Also, keep in mind that over washing hair can then cause the scalp to produce more oil (usually in younger people though), and this can clog follicles as well. Balance is needed to not "over strip" the hair/scalp of its natural oils. The use of certain liquid scalp cleansers that can be used before shampooing can really be helpful to use a few times per week to clean out hair follicles. When we use a 200x magnifying scope on clients to see changes in hair growth and thickness of strands, one of the first things we notice is cleaner follicles with regular use of these scalp cleaners or clarifying shampoos. This sets the stage for increased hair growth and thickness. There are also serums that aid hair growth that work by blocking DHT (with ingredients like Saw Palmetto), and also contain vitamins and minerals needed to feed the hair, which are great to use after the follicles get cleaned out weekly.

Another way to care for your scalp is to maintain scalp moisture and feed it good oils so it does not get dry. This can be done with the use of natural oils. Natural oils nourish the scalp and are a nice treat to massage in weekly, to aid in moisture and circulation to the follicles. Oil use will also bring nutrients contained in the oils to aid hair growth, add shine, and often strengthen the hair so it is less brittle, and there is less breakage and falling out. Some of the best oils to warm up and massage into the scalp are jojoba oil, coconut oil, sweet almond, castor, and olive oil. These can also serve as bases or "carrier" oil to essential oils for even more effect. A few drops of essential oil in 2-3 ounces of these carrier oils will enhance their effectiveness.

- Rosemary is a very good essential oil as it enhances circulation, and is a purifying and antiseptic agent that cleanses the hair follicles which is always helpful in aiding hair growth. This also aids in removal of any buildup, and stimulates the hair root to grow hair.

- Burdock oil which also works well for stimulating blood flow in the follicular roots, thereby helping in cell growth.

- Lemongrass oil helps to remove scalp buildup, and normalizes oil product in the scalp.

- Tea tree oil removes buildup on the scalp and helps rejuvenate dull hair.

- Peppermint oil can be used to energize and stimulate the scalp.

- Lavender essential oil has cell-regenerating properties. It can be used to promote hair growth and to prevent future loss.

- Sage is antiseptic and not only has an active agent to eliminate hair loss, but it strengthens and thickens the current hair shaft as well.

Debra Stoltzfus, nationally certified clinical aromatherapist and owner of Inshanti Essential Oils, states, "Therapeutically effective, quality, pure oils are expensive. Essential oils have become popular, and some companies take short cuts to reduce their costs. Make sure to purchase essential oils from a company that buys directly from the farmer/distiller, not from a marketing and distribution company or other 'middleman' that may cut or dilute the oils to increase profits. Oils should be stored in dark-colored glass bottles."

Her advice on a blend of oils that she uses in her practice for hair loss is, "Rosemary (Romarinus offincinalis) oil can stimulate the hair follicles, which results in hair growth. Jojoba Oil (Simmondsia chinensis) can loosen and remove buildup on the scalp that may block hair follicles and inhibit hair growth. Studies have shown that individuals suffering from alopecia (hair loss) who massaged their heads daily with lavender oil (Lavandula angustifolia) and other essential oils had significant hair re-growth over the course of seven months. When massaged into scalp, thyme oil (Thymus vulagarus ct. linalool) improves circulation, promoting the hair's shine, luster and bounce."

Laser Use to Stimulate Hair Growth and Health

Although the core of hair growth deals with nutrients and hormones, a large factor to get these nutrients, hormones, and oxygen to the hair follicles is blood supply. This is the one main focus of the topical solution on the market (*Minoxidol*). It would be very beneficial to increase micro- circulation to the scalp and hair follicles to aid this process and cause a synergistic effect to speed results. While fascia release and massage are a great start, lasers have been playing a role in this process of hair rejuvenation for years.

Laser light used in promoting hair growth is defined as Low-Level Laser Therapy (LLLT), or sometimes included under a broader definition of 'phototherapy', where a light-emitting device may be a laser and/or light-emitting diode (LED). The laser energy used to stimulate hair growth is visible in the red light spectrum. The first use of lasers was in Eastern Europe about twenty five years ago, to speed up the healing process of diseased people. Science has also supported since the late 1700s, that sunlight, or absence of it, directly affects the biochemistry of the body. Our hair is no exception to this.

Light affects how quickly our hair grows. We see evidence of this in our observation that our hair grows faster in the summer. This is simply due to improved blood supply to the hair follicles, stimulated specifically by the red light in sunlight.

Stated on the *Hair Loss Control Clinics* website, "A laser produces light measured at a wavelength of nanometers typical between 638.2 nM and 670 nM--a pure wave-length at the peak of red light in the visible light spectrum. Laser Hair Therapy light provides the essential boost of pure red light at precisely the right frequency to revitalize and repair hair, yet it utilizes a soft laser that uses less energy than a 40-watt light bulb."

Even a recent study released at the ISHRS Convention in Amsterdam, Netherlands 2009, presented by Dr. Grant Koher, called *"Effect of Laser Biostimulation In the Treatment of Female Pattern Hair Loss"* showed the following:

- 100% of the subjects saw an increase in hair growth

- 97% increased hair count equal to or greater than 20%

- 77% of the subjects increase of greater than or equal to 51%

There are many other long term international and recent clinical trials showing the benefits of lasers for hair growth stimulation. A European Study showed 100% retention of hairs and a 20% improvement in thickness and density of hair follicles using Laser Bio-Stimulation. A Laser received certification by the Canadian government for its ability to not only strengthen hair, but also prevent hair loss and stimulate re-growth in men and women.

I really like to combine therapies, so we have added a laser to our program for our clients to use in our center, or they may opt for a weaker, but still effective, hand-held unit for at home. Below is a list of what the laser specifically can do to aid hair loss:

- Speeds up/stimulates energy production in hair cells for optimal function and increases permeability of cell wall to nutrients.

- Increases protein synthesis for faster hair growth.

- Increases blood circulation to hair cells bringing nutrients to the cell, which increases the size of the actual capillaries feeding the hair cells.

If you are wondering what you can expect from the use of a laser, I can say, "It can seem slow, like waiting for grass for grow!" However, when it is "watered properly," hair responds faster. That is why the base levels of work need to be done first with stress and the hormones, as this is the reason the hair thinned to begin with. Then, it is smart to add in the laser and topical products which will then serve as the "icing" on the cake. Think of your hair as the icing on the "cake" of your body.

You want a good foundation to add the icing to, and that foundation, is hormone balance.

Based on years of experience from *Hair Loss Control Clinics,* with use of their larger in-house lasers 2-3 times per week, a client can experience faster hair growth, and the new hair will be more luxurious and manageable. When combined with proper scalp cleaning (as described), the scalp will have cleaner follicles which allow hair to grow efficiently. Soon clients notice more hair shafts growing per square inch, in about three to six months and that each individual hair strand is thicker in approximately six to nine months. Finally, more hair and thicker hair will be noticeable in the range of approximately eight to twelve months. Think of this type of therapy as a year commitment, but when you think of the return on your time, the investment it is well worth it.

Dietary Factor Foundation

When it comes to diet, the biggest component in our modern society connected to hair loss/thinning is increased sugar, or refined carbohydrate consumption. This increases "insulin resistance" over time, and will not only cause weight gain, but will decrease microcirculation to the hair follicle. In my opinion, from understanding hormones, decreasing overall sugar consumption is the best thing you can do in your diet for hair loss/ thinning. Coming up, we will discuss more foods that cause hair loss, and foods that help fight hair loss as somewhat of a dietary guide, but always keep in mind that any refined sugar is the enemy to eliminate!

Another bad American habit is consuming way too much caffeine, which will decrease vitamins, and therefore is not good for the hair either. The use of caffeine causes reactive hypoglycemia, and this will cause a blood sugar rollercoaster that indirectly increases cortisol and causes imbalances in sex hormones needed to prevent hair loss. Use of caffeine will also increase cravings as well, and guess what for....

SUGAR! Try to slowly lower caffeine and switch to something like green tea, which has less caffeine, or Yerba Mate tea, and even white or red (Rooibos) tea tastes great, containing no caffeine. These red and white teas also have some added flavors like peach, raspberry, or vanilla. Your hair and your central nervous system will thank you.

The other big issue in our country is that most people do not ingest enough protein, and hair and nails are made of protein. The formula for the amount of protein you should ingest per day is .8 grams of protein per kilogram of body weight. To help calculate this, a pound is 2.2 kgs so a woman weighting 150 lbs should have approximately 54.5 grams of protein per day. Increasing protein throughout the day will also aid in blood sugar stabilization, which stabilizes the stress hormone cortisol, allowing your sex hormones to balance. In order to aid protein digestion, it is wise to take digestive enzymes. Most people don't break down protein very efficiently after the age of twenty five. Digestive enzymes are like little "Pac Men" that break down proteins into the individual amino acids, to be used by the body for growth, maintenance, and repair. Protein does not get broken down until it reaches the stomach, and usually not very efficiently due to stress. A good digestive enzyme will also help break down fats, as well as carbohydrates - especially when you mix a lot of foods or eat heavy foods.

In America we can take more drugs than other countries. Another thing to keep in mind is that certain medications are connected to hair loss, they are:

- Blood thinners
- Psychotropic Drugs
- Pain Medications
- Synthetic Thyroid Medications
- Cholesterol Medications/Statins
- Birth Control Pill

This does not mean you should drop your medications immediately to make your hair grow, but this information could help you understand why you specifically might have a problem in this area, and it will be very important for you to do the other things that I mentioned in this chapter as well to help improve your hair growth.

Hormonal balance and the circulation of nutrients to hair follicle are the basis of healthy hair for men and women.

Foods that Help to Fight Hair Loss

Hair is affected by our nutrition, in that it is being fed by the blood supply carrying nutrients from the food we eat. This may seem obvious, but many people do not factor in nutrition - or what they eat or do not eat as playing a factor in their hair loss/thinning. The below information for foods that fight hair loss and foods that cause hair loss is taken from the Women Hair Loss Council 2009 Annual Report . You do not have to adopt all of these foods, or avoid all the harmful ones, but please read over these and see what foods you might be over eating or under eating that could help or hinder your hair loss/ thinning. This list can be used as a simple reverence or guide.

1. Yogurt: This is great for the hair due to its high Probiotic content, as well as its abundance of vitamin B-12, Magnesium, Potassium, and Calcium.

2. Sauerkraut: During the fermentation process, phytochemicals are produced. These are crucial because of their ability to aid during digestion. When choosing sauerkraut, be sure to choose one that is Organic (if possible), and one that is not pasteurized. The pasteurization process can kill all of the "good bacteria" that can benefit your digestive health.

3. Kombucha: This is a type of fermented probiotic tea. This works by being a natural adaptogen, meaning that it will work on a broad spectrum of imbalances within the body. It has been scientifically shown to boost energy, and detoxify the blood. You can find this in the health section of major grocery stores, as well as most health food stores.

4. Flax Seed: This is full of vitamins, and is the single highest source of lignans, which once in the intestines, will convert into a substance capable of balancing female hormones. This is great mixed in with yogurt, oatmeal, smoothies, cereals, and a variety of other foods.

5. Broccoli: As well as all of the vitamins that broccoli has, it also can help to balance blood pressure. It also contains some of the same phytochemicals, that we mentioned earlier, and because of the specific chemicals broccoli has the ability to destroy cancer causing agents. To maintain most of the benefits from broccoli, its best to steam it when cooking, and not boil it.

6. Beets: These contain Folic Acid which is very important in the health of your hair, as well as Phosphorus, Magnesium, Iron, and Potassium. Beets have the ability to detoxify your blood, and stimulate your liver and bile ducts to prevent artery disease.

7. Raw Ginger: Ginger contains an astonishing twelve different types of antioxidants. There's something called silica that's found in abundance in raw ginger, that actually fights hair loss. Taking silica in pill form will not help, it needs to be raw. Ginger can also help regulate women's menstruation cycles, and alleviate mild pain. For the best results, keep a piece of raw ginger in the fridge and cut off a small piece everyday and chew on it. You want to be sure you're getting brightly yellowed colored pieces and that the peel has been removed.

8. Garlic: Garlic contains something called allicin which has been proven to lower bad cholesterol (LDL). It is also capable of eliminating triglycerides in the blood. If there is a buildup of triglycerides in the blood, it can lead to a condition known as hypertriglyceridemia which is proven to negatively impact follicle size. Garlic is also best when it is eaten raw. For maximum results, try to eat at least four servings of garlic per week.

9. Cilantro: Fresh Cilantro is actually able to remove hormone disrupting heavy metals from your body, such as mercury and lead. There are many ways these metals find their way into our bodies. One major way is from fish, specifically tuna which is followed by shark, swordfish, marlin, lobster, cod, bass, and halibut. Silver dental fillings are another culprit, and also foods with high fructose corn syrup.

10. Green Tea: Researchers have found that green tea that contains catechin polyphenols is proven to not only fight cancer, but to

kill it without any damage to the healthy tissue. The reason I recommend green tea is that is does have some pick-me-up due to low caffeine content but not nearly as much as the blood sugar disturbing amounts in regular black tea or coffee.

11. Yerba Mate Tea: This is a calming tea that contains natural MAOI, meaning that it is a natural antidepressant due to it increasing dopamine. This tea also has less caffeine than black tea or coffee. Daily consumption of Yerba Mate Tea is just enough natural MAOI to decrease the symptoms of hypothyroidism so it can indirectly aid hair growth.

12. Nuts: Almonds, walnuts, pecans, hazelnuts, and cashews are all great to incorporate into your diet because of their higher levels of Omega-3 fatty acids which are essential in the health of hair follicles, and hair growth.

13. Lemon in Water: Drinking as little as one cup of lemon juice every morning over time has been shown to reset the bodies' chemistry and aid in keratinization, or hair growth.

14. Oranges and Tomatoes: Oranges and Tomatoes are full of many health benefits, one of them being their ability to strengthen our body's capillary walls. And it is our capillary walls that nourish and help strengthen our hair shaft because they lay right under the root of the hair follicle.

15. Olive Oil: When used in moderation in place of other fats, olive oil has been shown to lower cholesterol, and improve systolic blood pressure. As mentioned earlier increase of circulation, reduction of stress, and lower cholesterol all play a big role in the health of our follicles, and hair.

16. Fish Oil: There have been case studies proving the connection between fish oil, and the body's ability to hold onto newly grown hair. It has also been proven to actually strengthen the follicles themselves and not just the hair shaft.

17. Spices: Turmeric has been shown to aid in the recovery process of hair re-growth. It actually helps support nerve growth in the hair follicle itself. Cayenne reduces cardiovascular stress, which

correlates directly with stress levels and hair loss. Cinnamon is a blood sugar stabilizer and has the ability to lower the body's blood sugar without damaging the pancreas.

18. Eggs: Eggs are full of natural vitamins that stimulate follicles to promote growth, elasticity, and shine. A depletion of Vitamins A, E, B6, Copper, Iron, and Folate are reasons that America has such high rates of hair loss. One egg will provide 1/3 of these vitamins and consuming two eggs per day would cover your suggested amount of daily intake for these vitamins.

In conclusion on this section, try to use organic foods as often as possible because by eating organic, you are bypassing all of the toxic chemicals that non- organic foods are riddled with such as pesticides, chemical fertilizers, hormones, and antibiotics that will cause issues with your hormones.

Foods that Cause Hair Loss

1. Refined Sugars: As mentioned earlier in this chapter sugar is the key to "insulin resistance" and decreases micro-circulation and hormone disrupter. In addition, when your body is experiencing a rollercoaster of ups and downs with your insulin levels, it causes physiological stress, which leads to hair loss. An increase of insulin levels actually causes restriction on the release of your natural growth hormone (HGH) as well.

2. High Fructose Corn Syrup: Due to the way high fructose corn syrup is made it all contains small amounts of mercury as well as many other chemicals known for creating hair loss and causing hormone imbalances.

3. Sushi and other Fish: As we mentioned earlier, many fish, including tuna and salmon, have very high levels of mercury capable of disrupting our hormonal balance.

4. Dairy with RBST in it: (Recombinant Bovine Somatotropin). This is banned in many other countries but not the USA. RBST is a synthetic hormone that is injected directly into the dairy

cow responsible for making the milk they make our cheese, yogurt, etc to promote the growth of mammary glands so the cow produces more milk. Not only is this process extremely painful for the cow, it's also being put into our bodies through consumption, and is capable of causing cancer, which is why it is banned in other countries.

5. Meats containing sodium nitrates: Sodium nitrate is used to bleach fabrics, prevent metal corrosion, make rubber, and oddly enough to cure bacon. When cooked at higher temperatures this transforms into a compound capable of causing cancer. It will also wreak havoc on your hormones, cause migraines, and dramatically change your body's natural chemistry.

6. Alcohol: There have been many studies conducted on how much women's hair growth improves after cutting out alcohol, which is obvious to me, in that alcohol wreaks havoc on blood sugar and therefore disrupts hormones balance. Less known is that many people suffer from a slight allergy to alcohol that many times they do not know about and this indirectly will raise their cortisol levels.

7. Aspartame: Some call this "the most toxic substance on the market being sold to consumers," Aspartame has been to blame for over one million seizures in our country alone. Once ingested, Aspartame converts into formaldehyde and eventually leads to chronic formaldehyde poisoning, which will cause hair loss. Once you stop ingesting aspartame, it can take up to sixty days for your hair to start to re-grow.

In conclusion, avoiding processed food overall and eating real, whole foods will be key to hair health. In this process of switching over you will be also avoiding Genetically Modified Foods (GMOs) which are found in almost every processed food in the United States. Consuming genetically modified corn and soy is one of the leading reasons for health problems, including hair loss. Try to avoid eating foods that have corn or soy listed in its ingredients unless it says they are organic.

Additional Lifestyle Changes to Reduce Hair Loss

1. **Avoid excessive use of cell phones**: Cell phones emit radiation that affects the head and hair follicles. When using a cell phone, put it on speaker or use a headset. When you must hold it up to your ear, even holding it away an inch or two will decrease the amounts of radiation your hair follicles are absorbing.

2. **Non-stick Frying pans/ Teflon**: When Teflon is heated to high temperatures it releases toxic particles. Including one of the most toxic, PFOA, which causes hair loss and hair thinning. Replace Teflon coated pans with cast iron frying pans.

3. **Avoid Bpa/ Microwaved plastic**: BPA which is used in the production of most plastics and can leak into food and drink which will pose health hazards including hair loss. BPA can cause a hormone imbalance which is something our hair growth is heavily dependent upon. Limit taking in food and drink in plastic bottles and do not microwave anything in plastic.

4. **Household Cleaners:** Household cleaners are riddled with chemicals that can upset our hormones, which then can result in hair loss. There are many natural ways of cleaning your home without all of the harsh chemicals. Try replacing harsh chemicals with mixtures of vinegar, hot water, and baking soda for general household cleaning. Using essential oils to clean like Tea Tree oil is also a way to get great results without any harsh chemicals and you feel relaxed while you clean!

5. **Meditation:** Meditation is associated with strong hair shafts, follicles, roots and blood capillaries. Daily relaxation will decrease muscle tension of the scalp to also aid in fascia loosening. By meditating on a daily basis, you bring your body into homeostasis, which in turn makes the hair healthier and stronger by lowering cortisol and balancing hormones as mentioned. I recommend to my clients to do this daily, as a time of the day just for them, and to compensate for the overstimulation (even good stimulation) in our daily lives. An easy way is to start with a CD of sound waves and music

(possibly containing a voice-over). This will relax brainwaves patterns to the level of people who have trained for years in meditation. More information on this type of "sound wave" therapy can be found in Chapter 8.

6. **Inversion Therapy:** Laying on a slant board daily (anything where your feet are elevated at least 14 inches off the floor) will aid in increasing much needed blood to the head (great for the skin as well). This aids in bringing nutrients, hormones and oxygen to the scalp, which feeds the follicles and aids hair growth. You can do this while doing your daily 20 minutes of meditation or "sound wave" therapy to kill two birds with one stone. You will come out of this session very refreshed. Be cautious if you have high blood pressure or check with your doctor first.

7. **Relax Scalp/neck Muscles Regularly:** This can be done via massage to the neck or scalp yourself, from a loved one or a professional (perhaps monthly). The massage will lower your psychological stress, which directly lowers cortisol and aids hormone balance. It will also will increase circulation to the hair follicles. This will be even more effective if you have the fascia release done professionally first, if needed.

8. **Stimulation and Social Interaction:** By engaging in stimulating activity and social interaction, your body will release hormones (like dopamine and endorphins), which greatly stimulate hair growth and other positive reactions in the body.

9. **Have a Spiritual Connection:** Studies show people that pray or have a quiet time daily and believe in a higher power have lower stress hormones. Even though most Americas say they believe in a higher power, most do not take the time to "be still," and feel the presence of this power or to surrender to this power. I personally feel this daily quiet time lays a much better foundation for spiritual growth than church attendance. So if you are short on time, it is the most direct path to tapping into this "always accessible" power within you, and has my vote for priority.

Conclusion

Hopefully by reading this chapter, you can see that there are specific reasons for hair loss/thinning. Stress and hormones are always involved in hair health, and achieving natural hormone balance would be a great starting point for hair rejuvenation. It is not time passing (age), but abuse over time that will weaken parts of the body. In this case, this abuse weakens hair follicles, causing overall thinning and hair loss. The good news is that simple dietary and lifestyle changes outlined here can be adopted, and they will aid in the hormone balancing process. They also have many side benefits, such as improved mood, sleep, weight management and overall female health. The overall results will permeate more areas of your life than just your crowning glory that reflects back in the mirror!

TESTIMONIALS AND SUCCESS STORIES

T here are so many stories I would love to share on successful weight loss, improved mood, cessation of PMS and menopausal symptoms and increased vitality due to natural hormone balancing. I picked a few stories to share of the thousands we have seen and documented in our local center and across the country. The program and product(s) mentioned in these testimonials are all from the solutions mentioned in Chapter 8 of this book.

The names have been changed in these examples for privacy but this is not the preferred way I like to share testimonials. For some live video testimonials using actual full names, please see our website home page; and to see more written testimonials with names, click on the "testimonial" page of our website (BeBalancedCenters.com).

Relief from menopausal symptoms (insomnia, hot flashes/night sweats); avoiding synthetic HRT by utilizing progesterone and adrenal support in cream form.

"I would like to share with you how I am feeling since I started using the natural hormone balancing creams. I received my instructions, and within three days, I was sleeping through the night with no more night sweats. Now that my body has proper rest and has been balanced by the creams, I am on my way to healthy eating and weight loss, thirty pounds so far! I am very pleased with these creams, as I had not been able to lose weight in years."—Kim

"I had a complete hysterectomy four years ago and had been on HRT (estradiol). As the latest information became available for an increased risk in breast cancer and other complications (and I already have fibrocystic breasts) when on this, I went off this synthetic hormone and entered full- blown menopause. I then experienced severe night sweats, insomnia, hot flashes, and major hair loss as well as weight gain.

But when I started using natural hormone balancing creams, I seemed to balance out quickly! Though practicing daily in the medical field (nursing), I thank God for natural solutions."—Darla

"I began the natural hormone creams after I was in menopause. Previously, I had been on Vagifem for fifteen years, but when I learned of the consequences of excessive estrogen in the body, I was happy to make the switch. This week I had my annual OB/GYN exam, the first since being on the natural hormone creams. My doctor was very pleased with the condition of my vaginal tissue and encouraged me to keep using the natural hormone balancing creams. I am very pleased with these natural, simple-to-use products."—Nora

"I started the natural hormone balancing creams last April, and I could see a change in a few areas. First, I believe I slept better at night and second I didn't feel on edge during the day like I had. I even asked my OB/GYN what she thought about them and she said, *I'm starting to believe more and more that these products work.*' If anyone has a doubt, they should give them a try for themselves."—Sue

Relief from hormone imbalances causing severe pMS symptoms without the use of the birth control pill; utilizing progesterone and adrenal support in cream form.

Sara, age twenty-nine, came to us for some help with her hormones. She had been on the birth control pill for ten years to aid with severe menstrual cramps. After she had a stroke, she was advised to go off the birth control pill by her doctor and now was having severe PMS. She said she was not sure if the birth control pill was the cause of her stroke, but I reminded her that one of the side effects is a possible stroke. She started using the natural hormone balancing creams, and by her next cycle, she had no more menstrual cramps, irritability, or PMS. She was amazed that a natural solution could keep her symptoms under control with no side effects.

Rachael, age thirty-one, had come to us looking for answers as to why her symptoms of occasional seizures had come back after she had started on a micronized progesterone pill, which seemed to calm her and balance out her severe "estrogen dominance." A year ago she had brain surgery due to seizures that were uncontrollable even with medication. These started after being on the birth control pill for ten years for PMS symptom control and avoidance of pregnancy. She still had occasional seizures even after the operation and even with medication. At her latest doctor visit, her new OB/GYN suggested she get her hormones checked. She was found to be very low in progesterone and was given a micronized progesterone pill. For six to seven months afterward, she had no seizures at all and lowered her medication. But due to recent stress in her life, the seizures had returned. I explained it was probably due to her adrenal stress (not being addressed with the progesterone pill) and now the progesterone was being converted over to make cortisol. I also explained that due to stress her digestion was mostly likely less efficient and she should consider using a "trans-dermal" progesterone cream to bypass the digestive system for more efficient delivery. After she started both of the natural hormone balancing creams at a higher dosage, her seizures stopped again and she felt much better; we then cut her dosage back a bit. She kept monitoring her medications with her doctor hoping to get off of them altogether. Due to her severe hormone imbalance, we surmised the excitatory effect of estrogen would be implicated in her seizures and the brain surgery might have been avoided if she had her hormone levels checked first.

"I have suffered with stage-4 endometriosis for many, many years. ... I thought there must be something natural to help me. Thankfully, I found the natural hormone balancing creams, and I feel great! I stopped taking the birth control pill, and all of my monthly symptoms have been alleviated. No more water weight, irritability, breast tenderness, and other symptoms."—Janice

Relief from PMS, endometriosis, painful periods, fibroids and fibrocystic breasts; utilizing progesterone and adrenal support in cream form.

"I am thirty-two years old and was diagnosed with endometriosis and fibrocystic breast tissue in my early twenties. I wanted to rid myself of this issue and lose my last stubborn twenty or twenty-five pounds. I have battled severe periods—fevers, chills, diarrhea, heavy bleeding, and cramping so bad that I can't stand and must stay in bed with my heating pad. I started using the natural hormone balancing creams three weeks ago and just went through my last cycle since taking the creams. Wow! I only took one pain reliever the entire time! My body did not go through the typical symptoms (mentioned above) at all! The bleeding was much lighter, too. I also am down over twenty pounds that I was never able to lose before."—Robin

"I was having problems with bad PMS, headaches, irritability, bloating, and pain at ovulation. Within two cycles after starting on the natural hormone balancing creams I noticed a difference. No pre-ovulatory pain or migraine type headaches, etc."—Theresa

Diane came to my clinic to lose weight and balance her hormones. She started the weight loss program and did quite well over her two months reaching her goal weight. She also felt better due to the cessation of her PMS symptoms. She called me a few months later to let me know that the uterine fibroid that had been slowly growing was now completely gone. She had wondered if the program and her new hormone 'balance' had helped since her doctors were amazed. She then visited my center where we discussed this more and she showed me the doctor's reports. I assured her that her rise in progesterone due to her new hormone balance accounted for her estrogen no longer stimulating the fibroid to grow. She wanted to stay balanced so I put her on a natural progesterone cream for maintenance and some adrenal support in a cream form.

Relief from heavy bleeding and menstrual pain; avoiding an ablation utilizing progesterone and adrenal support in cream form.

Lisa, forty two, came to me out of desperation and after exhausting her patience with all her visits to doctors and specialists. She would bleed for three weeks straight, sometimes very heavy, each month for the last eight months. She could not take the birth control pill, a common "bandage" for this growing problem among pre-menopausal women. She did not want a hysterectomy and her ablation did not work. We started her on the natural hormone balancing creams as soon as she stopped bleeding. She then went into her very next cycle and went a full three weeks without her period and only started to menstruate the fourth week as normal. She went on using the natural hormone balancing creams monthly to maintain balance for a proper cycle and reported feeling much calmer and sleeping better.

Kathy, forty-six, started getting heavy, painful periods at age forty-four. The symptoms continued to worsen, so she decided to have an ablation as recommended by her doctor. She was not as concerned about lessening the flow as she was about easing the extreme pain she experienced every month. (Painful periods are common with annovulatory, or non-ovulating, menstrual cycles.) After the procedure, her flow decreased a bit, but the pain remained steady. Upon my recommendation, the following month she tried the natural hormone balancing creams I use in my center at the beginning of her cycle, and by time she got her period, it was much lighter and without pain. She was thrilled. She told me she plans to stay on the creams for an "improved quality of life."

Stubborn weight gone fast; Weight loss utilizing a low calorie ketogenic/glandular protocol

"While I was on a visit to Lancaster, PA in September of 2013, I was introduced to the Becoming Balanced...Hormonal Metabolic Correction Program at the local BeBalanced Center. At that time I was on bio-identical hormones (estrogen, progesterone and testosterone) for hot flashes and other menopausal issues but I gained weight and had sleep issues. I was not happy and was searching for something better. I eat well and do yoga and other exercise but still could not lose the belly fat. I started the Becoming Balanced program September 18, 2013. My weight was 140.5, and on October 30, 2013 I hit my goal weight of 120.5, a total of 20 lbs lost! The combination of the program's healthy diet, relaxation therapy and homeopathic blend helped me break through my weight loss barrier. The way I felt on the program, plus the step on the scale each day, gave me a lot of motivation, as the weight seemed to be melting away. I have recently been diagnosed with a Spinal Stenosis, and with the loss of belly fat the pain has been minimized. I feel that I have added years of renewed energy and good health. I feel better at 66 than I did at 50! --Suzanne

"By accident, I discovered the Becoming Balanced Program and thank God I did! Weight piled up on me after having an ovary removed. I tried different diets and joined a gym to take it off but to no avail - when you're a senior (age 59) it can be difficult! On the Becoming Balanced Program, I lost 39 lbs. in 6 weeks and went from a size 14 to a 6! My sugar cravings disappeared and I felt great inner peace - a benefit of natural hormone balancing. After more than a year, I'm still a size 6."—Kim

"I started in the Becoming Balanced...Hormonal Metabolic Correction Program and have lost 34 lbs. I always had problems losing weight. I felt it was my metabolism, but this was so easy! Also, when I would lose, it would not be from my rear end and hips. The Becoming Balanced program it triggered those areas, and I really lost there. I would tell anyone to try it! It works, I feel great! They are so helpful at The BeBalanced Center and that is a plus too! This was the best money I ever spent on myself!"—Ann

"I have been so grateful for this program. I have tried some other weight loss programs, but this program has been the only one that I lost weight on, and also felt absolutely fabulous inside and out! Feeling good inside meant I no longer had stomach problems (cramps, diarrhea). I have more energy now and no more night sweats. I noticed on the outside that even without exercise my body looks more toned. I have gone off multiple medications... it has just been amazing! I have told so many people about this program and how grateful I am that I have gone through it. Every time someone asks me how I did it I can't help but smile and gloat about your fantastic program. The best part is how natural it is and how wonderful it has made me feel. I can never thank the BeBalanced team enough for all of their encouragement through the process."—Debbie

"On the recommendation of a dear friend, I embarked on my journey of rediscovery. I reached a milestone birthday (50), and didn't like who I had become. I resigned from a poorly chosen career move and realized that the resulting obesity, stress, insomnia and irritability had to change or my health would soon decline. In October, I went to a BeBalanced Center and began the Becoming Balanced...Hormonal Metabolic Correction program. I faithfully followed the protocol, especially focusing on the relaxation elements. I am happy to say that not only have I lost 25 lbs, and lowered my cholesterol and my blood sugar (both down 10 points), I am stress free and sleeping soundly. I have added daily workouts and soothing meditation. I have a new love of healthy cooking and meal planning. I have a new sense of confidence knowing I can achieve anything I try. I like the new me so much more!"—Angie

"The Becoming Balanced...Hormonal Metabolic Correction program has helped me tremendously. I have lost 25 pounds faster than I ever thought possible, and I am cutting back on all my medications (for diabetes and my thyroid). My sleep has improved and I feel great overall with lots more energy and my stress level has decreased!"—Heather

"As I hit my forties I noticed I was struggling with keeping my weight steady. I was not sure what was causing this change in my body but after speaking with Dawn I realized I needed to balance my hormones. The Becoming Balanced Program has been very effective for me. I lost 25 lbs in 60 days, kept the weight off and maintaining my 116 lbs. I felt healthy, I looked great, people noticed, and my hips got smaller Yah! What I found even more remarkable was the cysts in my breast were gone. I would recommend this program to others".—Cindy

Thyroid stabilization/hormone balance with medication adjustments; utilizing a low calorie ketogenic/glandular protocol

"My TSH level in May 2010 was 3.6 and I was put on 88 mg of Synthroid; then my TSH level in December 2010 went up to 5.96, and I was raised to 100 mg of Synthroid. After only two months of doing the weight-loss program with natural hormone balancing, my TSH level in January 2011 was 2.3 (I was still on 100 mg of Synthroid), and I am now going to a lower dosage. The results may not be due solely to being on the program because my Synthroid medication was increased from 88 mcg to 100 mcg starting on December 9, however, I can say that my TSH levels have NEVER dropped that much with any increase in Synthroid medication including the first time I was diagnosed."—Emma.

"I remember initially deciding to look at the weight-loss program with natural hormone balancing after meeting with Dawn at the center and telling her, 'I'm desperate' with regards to needing to lose weight. Knowing myself, I needed a structured program to lose that thirty pounds I lost in the first round (month), but now I have signed up for a second round. I am looking and feeling better than I have in years! My thyroid medication has been decreased, and I am no longer dependent on my c-pap machine for sleep apnea! This program is changing my life!"—Cassandra

"I'm fifty-two years old and lost forty-five pounds on the weight-loss program with natural hormone balancing. I have been struggling with my weight since 1998 when my doctor discovered I had very low thyroid levels. Then in 2006, my thyroid was removed. After the surgery, my weight skyrocketed, and it was so hard to lose weight. I tried every diet out there. Nothing worked, until I sought professional help and found this unique program, which helped me lose the weight and keep it off. It helped me get off of blood pressure meds and lowered my thyroid medication. I have lots of energy, feel great about myself, really enjoy shopping for clothes, and love life in so many ways. I have learned how to eat healthy, which I share with my family every day. I highly recommend this program to anyone who is struggling with thyroid weight-gain issues."—Ilene

"I had been on a low dose of thyroid medication for eight years but still could not get my weight down to where it should be. After I started on the weight-loss program with natural hormone balancing, I felt really good, slept better and just felt calmer. About two to three weeks into the program, all of a sudden I started feeling agitated, I was not sleeping, and sometimes my heart would race. I was told this was due to my female hormones now having been balanced, that they were now allowing my thyroid to work more efficiently. I was advised to go to my doctor to get my thyroid medication dosage (Synthroid) checked. Sure enough, my TSH and T4 levels were showing my medication was too high, which would cause symptoms of being overmedicated. I ended up going off thyroid medication all together with my doctors help. Within a week I felt better and ended up losing twenty-one pounds that first month on the plan. I now understand how female sex hormone balance can positively affect the thyroid gland!"—Karla

Relief from mood issues of panic/anxiety and depression; Going off psychotropic drugs by utilizing progesterone and adrenal support in cream form.

"Since I started using natural hormone balancing creams, I do not have heart palpitations and I feel better. For years, I took medication for panic attacks. Now with the creams and relaxation CD, I have no need for my strong medication."—Kelly

"I have been using the natural hormone balancing creams almost 4 weeks. I have noticed that I am definitely less irritable and moody. I have also been able to go off my anti-anxiety agent. A reaction I did not expect was improvement in injection scars (from insulin injections) where I put the cream. Even my surgical scars are improving."—Julie

Debbie, thirty-six, came to us having been through a lot, emotionally, in her life, and she had also been on the birth control pill for over ten years to try to control her symptoms of severe PMS, depression, heavy periods, and weight gain that she could not lose (over thirty pounds in the last four years). She developed severe anxiety a few years back and had been put on Celexa. When her anxiety continued, she was constantly being put on more and more medication to control her panic attacks, which were not improving. She was prescribed Buspar, Diazepam, and then also Xanax as needed. She ended up being on three of each of these pills per day (along with her daily Celexa), a total of nine extra pills per day. After deciding to work with us on her hormones, our goal was to get the panic under control by increasing her progesterone levels. She began the natural hormone balancing creams for almost four weeks along with our relaxation CD daily and was able to wean herself from all nine of the extra pills (staying on her Celexa) giving her energy and zest for life back without the former panic attacks. She was going to then try to lose weight and wean off the final drug.

Relief from symptoms of aging (skin renewal, increased muscle response, increased libido and better sleep); utilizing HGH in a homeopathic form.

"I had lost thirty-five pounds on the weight loss program and was very happy. I wanted to go to the next level and really start getting fit with my new trimmer body. I started using the homeopathic HGH and started lifting weights to firm my muscles and add volume and firmness to my butt. I found my muscles responded so much better, like they did when I was in college! Even with adding some muscle weight I also lost 7 more pounds and now am a size 4!"—Katie

"I felt great after losing weight with natural hormone balancing. I was more confident, but wanted my skin to be a bit tighter under my arms and on my neck. I had combined the homeopathic HGH with some micro- current treatments and found the results to be synergistic. I was told that by stimulating the skin from the outside, the HGH worked even better as it stimulated skin renewal from the inside. I am very pleased with my results and plan to continue the HGH to slow down the aging of my skin!"—Karen

Helen felt great on the natural hormone balancing creams and reported her hot flashes had gone away and even her vaginal dryness was gone. She stated that she felt more energetic but still wished her libido would be a bit higher even though she enjoyed sex more now that her dryness issue was gone. After two months on the homeopathic HGH, Helen reported feeling much more zest for everything, like she was young and her sex drive increased to the point that it surprised her husband!

"I have been on the homeopathic HGH for about four weeks now, and I feel like I sleep so much deeper and wake up much more refreshed. I started to go to the gym in the morning now and feel energetic all day as a result."—Sheila

APPENDIX A

Lighten Up Emotionally Exercise

Underlying mental/emotional stress can take a toll on us long term and can disrupt our hormones. This is because it is almost like an upsetting event that keeps happening due to the fact that we cannot let it go.

Listed below are different areas where people tend to carry unresolved stress that they may look past or never think about. Please take time to think through and answer these questions on your own, perhaps during some quiet time over a cup of hot tea. When you pinpoint a few areas to work on, set up a specific time to relax in a prayer or meditative state and consciously "release" these emotions like balloons into the air.

All the issues we tend to hold on to, rob our daily energy since the body uses energy to hold on to them. Consider that your body has sixty watts of energy (like a light bulb) to run all of its systems every day. If you expend twenty to thirty watts worth of negative energy—thoughts like guilt, grudges, fears, and insecurities from past experiences—you only have thirty to forty watts of energy left to run your bodily functions, prevent deadly diseases (like cancer), and to focus on work, family, and spirituality. No wonder most of us are tired! There is not enough energy left to maintain all our needed functions and to run our body when we waste energy with negativity and stress.

As you aim for hormone balance, it is a good time to release pent-up emotions from your mind as well. As you correct and reset the body hormonally, you also need to correct faulty thinking patterns or limiting beliefs* as well as reset the way you think about your body, your relationships, and often, the world around you. This true renewing of your mind, body, and spirit will allow you to become all you were meant to be with nothing holding you back.

*Beliefs you hold as true in your mind that limit you in how you think and develop, or that keep you from reaching your full potential. (Examples of limiting beliefs are

"People are generally not helpful when I need it." "I never do well on tests." "I have never been able to keep my finances straight." "I always fail at losing weight.")

Childhood Traumas

Questions: Was anything in your childhood traumatic and perhaps still haunts you today?

Examples: Being stung by a bee, teased by kids for a specific reason, being scared of failing in school, death of a close family member, experiencing physical insecurity.

Parental Issues

Questions: Do you have unresolved feelings toward your parents whether they have passed away or are still alive?

Examples: Feeling like your parents did not really love you or did not love you unconditionally, feeling a high standard of perfectionism you felt insecure about living up to, still fearing parental criticism, dealing with loss/death of a parent, abandonment issues, resenting parental lack of discipline while growing up.

Self-Esteem Issues

Questions: Do you have feelings of anger, shame, or just insecurity due to something about yourself that needs to be altered?

Examples: Things that you do not like about your body, your personality, your mental skills, or your verbal skills.

Where You Are in Life Right Now

Questions: Are you living an authentic life, a life in alignment with who you are supposed to be on this earth, your purpose, and mission to serve humankind? Do you feel you are not where you should be in life right now, or not where you expected to be at this time? How do you feel about that? Are you resentful, angry, and fearful that things may never change? Do you feel like a powerless victim blaming everyone but yourself?

Examples: Currently hating your job or not feeling fulfilled daily from your work, wishing you were married by now or had children by this point in your life, feeling like you have no creative outlet that satisfies you, having little or no time to nurture yourself based on your overly busy schedule you have set for yourself.

The Importance of a Belief System

Having a strong belief system that gives you true comfort is really important. Most people have just adopted what their parents taught them and never questioned their beliefs. Often because of this, they are not in alignment with what their church denomination teaches. They just accept it because it is what the religious leader says. They are too busy to think any deeper about what they truly believe.

Most people never question or examine their beliefs because of fear. They may not have even looked around at other major faiths in the world to see the beauty and commonality with their own. They just dismiss other people's beliefs as wrong.

Questions: Do you feel alive in your faith? Are your beliefs rational by some standards? Do you accept that there are some things you will never know for sure but must accept by faith? Do you know that you can get most answers about your health, decisions in life, and more by meditating on your questions and praying? Do you feel your prayers and adopt a peaceful state while praying? Does your faith answer your questions of pain and suffering in the world and provide you comfort?

Examples: Accepting your parent's beliefs as your own and not feeling authentic in your profession of faith, feeling disconnected from God and therefore not loving yourself or others as you potentially could, fearing death and isolation it seems to bring, determining whether you fear judgment or God's wrath when you are not perfect or living up to some religious standards, feeling pressure to know what you believe when you feel abandoned by God or disillusioned by man's version of religion.

Coming to Terms with Love

Coming to terms with love and how to do it, feel it, and show it is a huge thing in life. After our basic needs of food, water, and shelter are met, love is perceived as the most important need.

Questions: Do you really feel loved by God, your spouse, friends, and children? Can you honestly say you have learned to love yourself? Do you feel like you know how to really love unconditionally?

If you answered "no" to any of these questions, work on loving yourself first and God and then you will be able to love others much better. Love is truly a capacity that can be learned. As you learn to love more it will be reflected back to you by those around you. The more you love the happier you will feel because you will feel more loved.

Day-to-Day Stress

Your day-to-day schedule is what you have created for yourself. It is a true reflection of your life on this earth. Not being happy and fulfilled daily in this schedule can cause many problems mentally and physically.

Questions: Do you feel rushed all the time? Do you have enough time to tend to your basic needs of bathing, exercise, and eating without rushing? Do you have a creative outlet daily or some free time to relax or read to stimulate your mind? Do you have time set aside for spiritual growth whether reading, praying, meditating or doing meditative exercises like yoga or Tai Chi? Is your emotional tank on empty at the end of the day because you gave to everyone else and have not been nourished yourself?

Conclusion

Now that you have spent time pinpointing areas of your life that you connect negative emotions to and then determining exactly what those emotions are, you are on your way to emotionally "lightening up." Next, just be willing and open to releasing them, which is the first step to letting them go. You must be willing to search your heart and soul and be honest with yourself. If you are ready, lay back and relax, and in your mind watch those balloons of negativity rise above your body and float away . . . never to be seen again.

APPENDIX B

Rejuvenation Center Study* on Progesterone Levels in Women with Hormone Sensitive Cancers; Oct 2009

This study has now since been published in the September 2012 edition of the *Original Internist.*

The study set forth in this appendix was done over a two year span by hormone specialist Joseph Beldonza C.C.N, who has performed over 20,000 saliva hormone tests and who educates doctors on a national level on hormones. The study took place at the Rejuvenation Center in Lancaster, PA and was facilitated by the center owner holistic health practitioner, Dawn M. Cutillo. Bio Health Lab from California evaluated the saliva test and Dr. Lorraine Bernotsky, research director, West Chester University, West Chester, PA, tabulated the study results.

*Now the first BeBalanced Center

Details of the Study Sample:

A group of 25 local women who have had breast cancer in the last 5 years (not currently on chemotherapy, radiation or medication) were compared to a group of 20 women who never had breast cancer.

Goal of the Study:

To show trends in saliva hormonal profiles of women who have had breast cancer. These trends could then serve to aid women who want to prevent breast cancer by allowing them to compare their saliva test results to these in an effort to early detect the possible manifestation of the disease.

Main Findings of the Study:

- Low levels of progesterone are linked to breast cancer

- High levels of estrogen (estradiol) in relation to progesterone (an imbalance) is linked to breast cancer

- More research is worth pursuing to see specific ratios of the three main estrogens and breast cancer occurrences

These are interesting findings not often brought to women's attention. Although biomedical literature recognizes the importance of the relationship between progesterone levels and the incidence of breast cancer, mainstream medical practice does not. However, some medical professionals have investigated and tracked this relationship in their own patients (see for example, Dr. John R. Lee's work) and have suggested that the use of estrogen therapy to address symptoms of menopause puts patients at risk with respect to decreased levels of progesterone. In fact, the American Cancer Society's webpage does not differentiate between estrogen and progesterone when citing hormones that could be related to the incidence of breast cancer. In this manner, it would seem that traditional medical opinions do not recognize or emphasize the potentially important role of progesterone in women's health, including breast cancer among various other health concerns.

This study emphasizes the known fact that women with breast cancer have a hormonal imbalance.

Details of the Study:

There appears to be a relationship between the incidence of breast cancer and progesterone levels when comparing the 25 women with breast cancer to 20 similarly-aged women who never had breast cancer. All of the women with breast cancer had low progesterone levels, as far as Mr. Beldonza reports, based on his evaluation of "normal/healthy" levels.

But when comparing the cross-sample of 45 women over 69% of women with extremely low levels of progesterone (under 100) had breast cancer, while only 42.9% of those with slightly higher levels of progesterone (over 100) Had breast cancer. It is important to note that those with levels over 100 still were low overall—but the lower the progesterone the increased risk of breast cancer.

This is compounded by the relationship between the incidence of breast cancer and the ratio of progesterone to estradiol (an estrogen) when comparing women with ratios under 50 to those with ratios over 50. The study showed that 73.1% of women with progesterone to estradiol ratios lower than 50 had breast cancer, while only 31.3% of those with ratios over 50 had breast cancer.

More interesting was the trends in the specific levels and ratios of the three estrogens tested, though this requires further research. It was found that 64% of these women had an estradiol level lower than their estrone level. Almost all women (96%) had an estriol level that was lower than their estradiol level while 76% had an estradiol level that was different by less than 1 point from their estriol level. "While not being statistically significant at this point, this finding is worth further research" reports Dr. Bernotsky as she tabulated the results.

Conclusion:

More research is needed into the exact estrogen profiles but a strong link exists between progesterone levels and breast cancer as well as the ratios of high estradiol to progesterone levels as an indicator of breast cancer.

Balancing estrogen and progesterone levels naturally before breast cancer can develop would be Mr. Joseph Beldonza's advice to women who fear developing the disease. Some symptoms of "estrogen dominance" (which indicates an imbalance of estrogen and progesterone) are PMS, depression, anxiety, irritability, insomnia, headaches, hot flashes, mood swings, strong food cravings, fluid retention, etc.

Joe Beldonza is a certified clinical nutritionist (C.C.N.) and has been in the health field since 1981. He is a doctor of naturopathy and additionally has graduated from over fifty courses in the health care field; some of which are: Nutrabalance Blood Chemistry Assessment, Environmental Stress Management, Homeopathic Solutions, Bradford Research Institute Blood Chemistry, and Sabre Sciences Hormone

Analysis Research. His diversities include: General Nutrition, Homeopathic, Herbology, Live Blood Analysis, and Diagnostics. He has personally analyzed over 20,000 hormone tests and helped start a major hormone testing lab. Mr. Beldonza has been educating doctors, chiropractors and other health care professionals on how to utilize nutrition for patient care to enhance the effects of their daily practice.

APPENDIX C

Studies on hCG and Weight Loss

Removed from 2nd edition of The Hormone Shift

This section is no longer applicable as Dawn, through her BeBalanced Centers, switched from the usage of homeopathic hCG to a homeopathic glandular blend combined with a low calorie ketogenic diet plan as noted in Chapter 3.

APPENDIX D

Statistics for Clients on a Low-Calorie Ketogenic Diet

The table below shows typical weight loss statistics from twenty five clients using the Becoming Balanced...Hormonal Metabolic Correction program (taking a homeopathic formula utilizing hCG) in a thirty day protocol. This table is used to show that by utilizing the Simeons hCG protocol, fat loss is a high percentage of overall *weight loss*. This in turn will yield the preservation of lean muscle mass, not typical with normal low calorie diets. Dawn, through BeBalanced Centers, has now changed to a low calorie ketogenic/glandular protocol to replace hCG now that it is off the market. This same principle of *fat* loss (as opposed to muscle loss) will apply to the new low calorie ketogenic/glandular protocol so therefore this Appendix was left in the second edition. The below chart will show that when hormones are balanced and a ketogenic state is achieved by the body, there is no catabolic (muscle loss) effect.

First name	Round 1 Body Fat % Loss	Round 1 pounds lost	Round 1 Fat pounds lost	Round 1 Inch loss
Claudia	6.20%	16.8	16	14.5
Sue	2.60%	25.6	20.2	12.25
Tana	5.60%	17.6	14.6	12.5
Lori	6.70%	20.2	16.6	16.25
Rebecca	10.60%	23.4	17.8	20.25
Susana	4.10%	14	11	11.5

First name	Round 1 Body Fat % Loss	Round 1 pounds lost	Round 1 Fat pounds lost	Round 1 Inch loss
Randy	5.80%	22.8	16	12.5
Linda	4.40%	28.4	20.2	16.25
Diane	3.00%	26.2	22.4	13
Amy	3.60%	23.8	19.4	11
Maryln	1.40%	15.4	10.4	8.5
First name	Round 1 Body Fat % Loss	Round 1 pounds lost	Round 1 Fat pounds lost	Round 1 Inch loss
Sara	2.00%	16.6	7.4	8
Barbara	0.70%	16.8	9.6	12.5
Rick	2.60%	28.6	17	14
Diane	4.00%	20.6	15.6	17.75
Cathy	4.10%	19.2	13.4	15.75
Jennifer	0.80%	20.6	11	14.75
Jenn	1.20%	21.4	8.6	12
Cindi	2.10%	23.8	14.6	12.25
Angela	7.10%	19.6	17.4	15.75
Kristi	1.30%	12.8	8.8	15.5
Deb	4.90%	18	12.8	17.75
Barb	2.40%	18.2	15.8	14
Deb	5.90%	17	15.2	12
Jennifer	4.50%	20.4	19.4	18

APPENDIX E

Classifications of Major Classes of Birth Control Pills

1st Generation Progestin

<u>BR ANDS</u>: *Ortho -Novum, Estrostep Fe, Zovia, Demulen, Loestrin, Demulen, Loestrin, Estrostep Fe, Aygestin, Camila, Errin, Jolivette, Nor-QD, Nora-Be, Ortha Microvior, Aranelle, Balziva, Femcon Fe, Jenest-28, Junel, Microgestin, Modicon, Necon, Orcon 35, Rilia FE, Zenchent, Nortel, Tri-Norinyl, Tri-Legest Fe*

Names of the progestin: Norethindrone, Norethindrone Acetate, Ethynodiol Diacetate

This form has:
- low to medium progestational activity
- slight estrogenic activity
- tends to be less androgenic

<u>Positive Effects:</u> This progestin improves lipid profiles by raising HDL and lowering LDL; may be helpful for women who experience minor estrogen- related side effects such as nausea, migraines, or fluid retention with other pill combinations.

<u>Side Effects:</u> Tends to be associated with increased early or midcycle breakthrough bleeding and spotting as compared to other combination pills; often higher estrogen dosages will be used with this progestin to counteract the likelihood of breakthrough bleeding. Therefore, pill brands that contain higher levels of estrogen can alleviate this side effect.

2nd Generation Progestin

BR ANDS: *Seasonique, Mirena, Alesse, Aviane, Lessina, Levien, Levora, Lutera, Lybrel, Nordette, Portia, Sronx, Enpresse, Levlite, Tri-Levan, Triphasil, Trivora, Jolessa, LeSeasonique, Quasense, Seasonal, Orvette, Cryselle28, Low-Ogestrel, Ogestrel, Ovral, Lo/Ovral*

Names of the Progestin: Levonorgestrel, Norgestrel This form has:

- high progestational activity

- high androgenic effects

- sometimes strong anti-estrogen effects

Positive Effects: This progestin improves estrogen-related side effects such as nausea, migraines, or fluid retention often found with using other pill combinations that have higher estrogenic activity.

Side Effects: This progestin negatively affects serum lipoproteins; it may cause LDL cholesterol to be increased while allowing for HDL cholesterol to be lowered

3nd Generation Progestin

BR ANDS: Cyclessa Triphasic Pill, Ortho Tri-Cyclen Lo, NuvaRing, Implanon, Mononessa, Ortho Cyclen, Orth Tri-Cyclen, Tri-Previferm, Tri- Sprintec, Trinessa, Ortho Evra (the Patch)

Names of the progestin: Norgestimate, Etonogestrel, Desogesterel This form has:

- high progestational selectivity

- minimal androgenic effects and estrogenic activity

- some have slight estrogenic effects.

Positive Effects: It shows less negative impact (but still some!) on metabolism, weight gain, acne, and other side effects typical of older progestin; has been used for the successful treatment of acne; also has minimal effect on serum lipoproteins as well as on carbohydrate metabolism; may be helpful in lowering side effects such as nausea and vomiting while not causing an increased incidence of spotting (typically associated with low-estrogen, high progestin pills).

Side Effects: Clinical trials show a potential for a higher risk of nonfatal venous thrombosis

4th Generation Progestin

BRANDS : *Angeliq, Yasminelle, Yaz, Yasmin, Ocella*

Names of the progestin: Drospirenone, Dienogest, Nesterone, Nomegestrel, and Trimegestone

This form has:

- High progestational effects
- Minimal androgenic effects Derived from 17a-spirolactoneis.

Positive Effects: This form has a pharmacological profile which more closely mimics natural progesterone. It also has low androgenic activity; treats acne in females; may cause fewer hormone fluctuations than typical BC pills.

Side Effects: It helps suppress the secretion of the hormones that regulate the body's water and electrolytes, which can potentially cause hyperkalemia in high-risk patients. Hyperkalemia is a condition in which the concentration of potassium (K+) in the blood is elevated. Extreme hyperkalemia is a medical emergency due to the risk of potentially fatal abnormal heart rhythms (arrhythmia); contraindicated in patients with hepatic dysfunction, renal insufficiency, adrenal insufficiency.

Because of the anti-mineralocorticoid effects, care needs to be exercised when other drugs are used that may increase potassium levels (examples NSAIDS which are common and ACE inhibitors, potassium-sparing diuretics, potassium supplementation, heparin, aldosterone antagonists).

APPENDIX F

Classes of Psychotropic Medications / Withdrawal Side Effects

If you are on a psychotropic drug, see if you can find yours on this list so you can better understand what action it has on the body. Then, the next section will aid you in seeing the possible side effects of weaning off (with your doctor's help).

Examples of the Classes of Psychotropic Medications

The major Antidepressants, MAOI, SNRI, SSRI, Tricyclics, Antipsychotics and Anti-Anxiety medications are broken down for you in the list below to help you understand the different categories (classes) of psychotropic medications.

1. Antidepressants (Atypical)—They are each unique medications that work in different ways from one another. Atypical anti-depressants ease depression by affecting chemical messengers (neurotransmitters) used to communicate between brain cells.

    *   *Trazadone, Remeron, Wellbutrin, Serzone, Ludiomil*

2. MAOI—Work to prevent an enzyme that breaks down serotonin, melatonin, epinephrine and norepinephrine (to increase their availability in the brain). More side effects occur with this class of drug than standard SSRI or SNRI drugs but often used when these classes of drugs will not provide relief of symptoms.

    *   *Manerix, Marplan, Nardil, Parnate*

3. SNRI—Work to inhibit the reuptake (or reabsorbing) of Serotonin and Norepinephrine

    - *Cymbalta, Effexor*

4. SSRI—Work to inhibit the reuptake (or reabsorbing) of Serotonin

    - *Celexa, Lexapro, Luvox, Paxil, Prozac, Symbyax, Zoloft*

5. Trysiclics—An older form of antidepressant drug named after its molecular shape that works to inhibit the reuptake of both Serotonin and Norepinephrine; the therapeutic dose is close to a toxic dose hence these drugs are used less and replaced by newer SSRIs and SNRIs.

    - *Amitriptyline, Amoxapine, Clomipramine, Desipramine, Trimpramine*

6. Typical Antipsychotics—Work to block receptors in the brain's dopamine pathways, but antipsychotic drugs encompass a wide range of receptor targets as well; first generation; developed before "atypical" forms.

    - *Haldol, Loxitane, Mellaril, Moban, Navane, Orap, Thorazine, Trilafon*

7. Atypical Antipsychotics—Work to block receptors in the brain's dopamine pathways, but antipsychotic drugs encompass a wide range of receptor targets as well; second generation, developed more recently than "typical" form. Atypicals are thought to cause fewer serious or long term side effects.

    - *Abilify, Clozaril, Geodon, Risperdal, Seroquel, Zyprexa*

8. Anti-Anxiety/Benzodiazepines—Work to enhance the effect of the neurotransmitter (GABA) gamma-aminobutyric acid. The result is sedation or a hypnotic (sleep-inducing) effect and can produce an anxiolytic (anti-anxiety) or anticonvulsant effect. Usually used to treat anxiety, insomnia, or agitation when in

reference to mood stabilization; they are either shorter or longer acting and prescribed based on the action needed. This class of medication is one of the more frequently prescribed for panic or anxiety disorders.

- *Serax, Klonopin, Xanax, Ativan, Librium, Valium*

Withdrawal Effects of Mood Stabilizing Medications

Below are a few examples to show you the complications of weaning off a psychotropic drug. You should only attempt to slowly wean off these medications with your doctor's help. It may be helpful to ask your doctor if you can get your medication in a liquid form at a local apothecary so that is easier to wean off of in a slow systematic way. Depending on the medication, some can take as long as 2-3 months to wean off of safely with no withdrawal symptoms.

These below stated symptoms have been taken directly from the pharmaceutical companies packaging and warnings.

Effexor (SnRI)—requires a gradual reduction in the dose rather than an abrupt cessation, whenever possible, to avoid withdrawal symptoms that include: agitation, anorexia, anxiety, confusion, impaired coordination and balance, diarrhea, dizziness, dry mouth, dysphoric mood, fasciculation, fatigue, flu-like symptoms, headaches, hypomania, insomnia, nausea, nervousness, nightmares, sensory disturbances (including shock-like electrical sensations), somnolence, sweating, tremor, vertigo, and vomiting. *This medication should be weaned off SLOWLY and GRADUALLY.*

Cymbalta (SnRI)—has a very short half life (only 12 hours), so withdrawing suddenly can cause a variety of undesired symptoms such as headaches, brain "shivers," constant nausea and flu-like symptoms (vomiting, fever chills, sore throat, diarrhea) and even seizures. *This medication should be weaned off of SLOWLY and GRADUALLY.*

Zoloft (SSRI)—has a half-life of about 24 hours. If a patient stops Zoloft too rapidly a withdrawal syndrome may develop. Among the symptoms that may be experienced are nausea, tremors, lightheadedness, muscle pain, weakness, insomnia and anxiety. The withdrawal symptoms usually last 1-2 weeks but in some cases they may gradually decrease over a period as long as one month. *It is recommended that a patient taper off this medication SLOWLY and GRADUALLY.*

Prozac, Paxil, Lexapro (SSRI)— these drugs have been reported to cause adverse events upon their discontinuation (particularly when abrupt), including the following: Dysphoric mood, irritability, agitation, dizziness, sensory disturbances (e.g., paresthesias such as electric shock sensations and tinnitus), anxiety, confusion, headache, lethargy, emotional stability, insomnia, and hypomania. While these events are generally self-limiting, there have been reports of serious discontinuation symptoms such as seizure. *A GRADUAL REDUCTION in dose rather than an abrupt cessation is recommended whenever possible.*

Xanax (anti anxiety-benzodiazapine)— abruptly stopping or cutting down on your prescribed dosage may cause a spectrum of discontinuation symptoms that can be unpleasant and even dangerous; the most important is seizure. Other more common discontinuation symptoms of Xanax include tremor, headache, insomnia, nervousness, diarrhea, depression, and decreased appetite. *This medication should be weaned off of SLOWLY and GRADUALLY.*

Ativan (anti anxiety-benzodiazapine)— a highly addictive class of drugs; long term effects of using this class of drug are tolerance, dependence, and cognitive impairments which may not completely reverse after cessation of treatment. Withdrawal symptoms can range from anxiety and insomnia to seizures and psychosis. Adverse effects including anterograde amnesia, depression and paradoxical effects such as excitement or worsening of seizures may occur. *This medication should be weaned off of SLOWLY and GRADUALY.*

APPENDIX G

Homeopathy Described

Homeopathy is a type of alternative medicine that has been used in our country since the European settlers came to America. The basic principle of homeopathy is "let like be cured by like." Dr. Martin Chaplin, an Emeritus Professor of Applied Science at the London South Bank University, explains homeopathy to be "a branch of alternative medicine that is based around the surmise that an individual may be treated using minute doses of natural materials which in larger doses would be expected to cause the same symptoms. Remedies are made by a sequence of dilutions of the starting material in purified water or aqueous ethanol with considerable agitation (called succussion)."

When writing for the Huffington Post, Dana Ullman—an expert in homeopathic medicine—states, "One metaphor that may help us understand how and why extremely small doses of medicinal agents may work derives from present knowledge of modern submarine radio communications. Normal radio waves simply do not penetrate water, so submarines must use an extremely low-frequency radio wave. The radio waves used by submarines to penetrate water are so low that a single wavelength is typically several miles long!"

If one considers that the human body is seventy to eighty percent water, perhaps the best way to provide pharmacological information to the body and into intercellular fluids is with nanodoses. Like the extremely low-frequency radio waves, it may be necessary to use extremely low (and activated) doses for a person to receive the medicinal effect.

It is important to understand that nanopharmacological doses will not have any effect unless the person is hypersensitive to the specific medicinal substance. Hypersensitivity is created when there is some type Of resonance between the medicine and the person. Because the system of homeopathy bases its selection of the medicine on its ability to cause the similar symptoms that the sick person is experiencing, homeopathy's principle of "similars" is simply a practical method of finding the substance to which a person is "hypersensitive."

In homeopathy, a substance such as a drug, steroid, herb, or vitamin is diluted down several times in distilled water (with alcohol to stabilize it) and is noted as dilutions of 1x, 2x, 3x . . . 100x. The more diluted the substance the less "strong" it is and the fewer "side effects" it would have (if it were a drug originally being used). However, its vibration would be raised and it would have a more powerful effect on the body. The National Center for Complementary and Alternative Medicine explains this even further by stating, "The principle of dilutions (or 'law of minimum dose') states that the lower the dose of the medication, the greater its effectiveness. In homeopathy, substances are diluted in a stepwise fashion and shaken vigorously between each dilution. This process, referred to as 'potentization,' is believed to transmit some form of information or energy from the original substance to the final diluted remedy. Most homeopathic remedies are so diluted that no molecules of the healing substance remain; however, in homeopathy, it is believed that the substance has left its imprint or 'essence,' which stimulates the body to heal itself (this theory is called the 'memory of water')."

In my opinion, these formulations are safer (most have no documented side effects) but are just as effective, and sometimes even more effective than the original drug substances due to the fact that they do not tax the liver and do not stress the body with side effects. While most prescription drugs treat the symptoms of a disease, homeopathy is intended to treat the root of a problem rather than the symptoms. Homeopathy looks to find the cause of the symptoms, which often has to do with subtle imbalances in the system. These imbalances, as you've learned, are sometimes hormonal. Homeopathy promotes healing and strengthening in the body and helps to restore balance.

I use a homeopathic form of HGH in my center for its anti-aging effects and a homeopathic glandular with our low-calorie ketogenic diet.

References:

Martin, Chaplin, Dr. (2011, October 31). Water Structure and Science: Homeopathy. Retrieved from http://www.lsbu.ac.uk/water/homeop.html.

Ullman, Dana. (2009, December 12). How Homeopathic Medicines Work: Nanopharmacology at its Best. Huffpost Healthy Living. Retrieved from http://www.huffingtonpost.com.

REFERENCES

CHAPTER 1

Lee, John R., Jesse Hanley, and Virginia Hopkins. (1999). *What Your Doctor May Not Tell You about Pre-menopause.* New York: Grand Central Publishing.

Lee, John R. and Virginia Hopkins. (2004). *What Your Doctor May Not Tell You about Menopause.* New York: Wellness Central.

Lee, John R. and Virginia Hopkins. (2006). *Hormone Balance Made Simple.* New York: Grand Central Life & Style.

Randolph, C.W., Jr., M.D. & James, Genie, M.M.Sc. (2009). *From Hormone Hell to Hormone Well: Straight Talk Women (and Men) Need to Know to Save Their Sanity,Health, and—Quite Possibly— Their Lives.* Deerfield Beach, Fl: Health Communications, Inc.

Schwartz, Erika, M.D. (2002). *The Hormone Solution: Naturally Alleviate Symptoms of Hormone Imbalance from Adolescence through Menopause.* New York, NY: Warner Books, Inc.

Stanton, Alicia, M.D. and Tweed, Vera. (2009). *Hormone Harmony.* Los Angeles, CA: Healthy Life Library.

Wiley, T.S. and Bent Formby. (2000). *Lights Out: Sleep, Sugar, and Survival.* New York: Pocket Books.

Wilson, James L. (2001) *Adrenal Fatigue: The 21st Century Stress Syndrome.*Petaluma, CA: Smart Publications.

CHAPTER 2

Allen, Loyd V., Jr. (2008). Estriol: Women's Choice vs. A Manufacturer's Greed. *International Journal of Medicine,* 1212(4), 289.

Arpels, JC. (1996). The Female Brain Hypoestrogenic Continuum from the Pre-menstrual Syndrome to Menopause [Abstract]. *Journal of Reproductive Medicine,* 41(9), 633-639.

Asplund, R. and Aberg, H. (1996). Nocturnal Micturition, Sleep and Well-Being in Women of Ages 40-64 Years [Abstract]. *Maturitas,* 24, 73-81.

Casper, R.F., Yen, S.S.C. and Wilkes, M.M. (1979). Menopausal Flushes: A Neuroendocrine Lnked with Pulsatile Luteinizing Hormone Secretion [Abstract]. *Science,* 205, 83-93.

Cowan, L.D. et al. (1981, August). Breast Cancer Incidence in Women with a History of Progesterone Deficiency. *American Journal of Epidemiology,* 114(2), 209-217.

Grady, Deborah, et al. (2003). Predators of Difficulty When Discontinuing Postmenopausal Hormone Therapy. *Obstetrics and Gynecology,* 102(6), 1233-1239.

Huerta, R., et al. (1995). Symptoms at the menopausal and pre-menopausal years: their relationship with insulin, glucose, cortisol, FSH, prolatin, obesity and attitudes towards sexuality [Abstract]. *Psychoneuroendocrinology,* 20(8), 851-864.

Lee, John R., Jesse Hanley, and Virginia Hopkins. (1999). *What Your Doctor May Not Tell You about Pre-menopause.* New York: Grand Central Publishing.

Lee, John R. and Virginia Hopkins. (2004). *What Your Doctor May Not Tell You about Menopause.* New York: Wellness Central.

Lee, John R. and Virginia Hopkins. (2006). *Hormone Balance Made Simple*. New York: Grand Central Life & Style.

Randolph, C.W., Jr., M.D. & James, Genie, M.M.Sc. (2009). *From Hormone Hell to Hormone Well: Straight Talk Women (and Men) Need to Know to Save Their Sanity, Health, and—Quite Possibly—Their Lives*. Deerfield Beach, Fl: Health Communications, Inc.

Reiss, Uzzi. (2001). *Natural Hormone Balance for Women*. New York: Pocket Books.

Stanton, Alicia, M.D. and Tweed, Vera. (2009). *Hormone Harmony*. Los Angeles, CA: Healthy Life Library.

Thurston, R.C., et al. (2008, May-June). Abdominal adiposity and hot flashes among midlife women. *Menopause, 15*(3), 429-434.

Vom Saal F, Hughes C. (2003). An extensive new literature concerning low- dose effects of bisphenol A shows the need for a new risk assessment. *Environmental Health Perspectives, 111*, 926-933. See: http://www.ehponline.org/members/2005/7713/7713.html

Wiley, T.S. and Bent Formby. (2000). *Lights Out: Sleep, Sugar, and Survival*. New York: Pocket Books.

Wilson, James L. (2001) *Adrenal Fatigue: The 21st Century Stress Syndrome.* Petaluma, CA: Smart Publications.

Zavik, Jeffrey S. and Thompson, Jim. (2002). *Toxic Food Syndrome*. Ft. Lauderdale, FL: Fun Publishing.

CHAPTER 3

Annette Copeland, CNHP. "A Study to Determine the Effectiveness of Homeopathic Weight Loss Remedies: HCG ~vs~ non-HCG." *The Original Internist* Volume 18. Issue 3 (2011): 107. Print.

Kossoff, E.H., et al. (2009 Aug). Ketogenic diets: an update for child neurologists. *J Child Neurol*, 24(8), 979-988.

Shute, N. (2011, Dec 28). Could Obesity Change The Brain? Retrieved from http://www.npr.org/blogs/health/2011/12/27/144331177couldobesity-change-the-brain.

Simeons, A.T.W. (1976). Pounds and Inches: *A New Approach to Obesity*. Private Printing.

Simeons, A.T.W. (1954). The Action of chorionic gonadotrophin in the obese. *Lancet II*, 946-947.

https://umm.edu/health/medical/ency/articles/hypothalmis-dysfunction

http://www.news-medical.net/news/20131106/normal-blood-suagrregulation-depends-on-partnership-between-pancreas-and-brain.aspx

http://www.nejm.org/doi/full/10.1056/NEJM199309303291401#t=article

www.health-matrix.net/2013/08/09/the-ketogenic-diet-an-overview/

http://selfgrowth.com/articles/are-your-major-hormones-in-balanceinsulin-and-cortisol-balance

http://www.ncbi.nlm.nih.gov/pmc/articles/PMC2367001

http://www.ketogenic-diet-resource.com/ketogenic-diet-benefits.html

http://ncbi.nlm.nih.gov/pubmed/15148063

http://www.pethealthandnutritioncenter.com/kidney-glandularsupplement-from-new-zealand.html

http://www.vcahospitals.com/main/pet-health-information/
articleanimalhealth/supplements-whole-food-supplements/575*

* This client information sheet is based on material written by: Steve Marsden, DVM ND MSOM LAc DiplCH AHG, Shawn Messonnier, DVM and Cheryl Yuill, DVM, MSc, CVH

CHAPTER 4

Arem, Ridha, M.D. (2008). *The Thyroid Solution: The Doctor-Developed, Clinically Proven Plan to Diagnose Thyroid Imbalance and Reverse Thyroid Symptoms.* Rodale, Inc.

Benson, Herbert et al. (1975). *The Relaxation Response.* New York: Avon (reissue 1990).

Benson, Herbert and Proctor, William. (1984). *Beyond the Relaxation Response.* New York Times Books.

Chopra, Deepak. (1990). *Quantum Healing.* New York: Bantam Books.

Erdmann, Robert and Jones, Meirion. (1995). *Fats that Can Save Your Life.* Port Orchard, WA: Bio-Science.

Kharrazian, Datis, D.H.Sc., D.C., M.S. (2010). *Why do I Still Have Thyroid Symptoms?* Garden City, NY: Morgan James Publishing, LLC.

Lee, John R. and Virginia Hopkins. (2004). *What Your Doctor May Not Tell You about Menopause.* New York: Wellness Central.

Lee, John R. and Virginia Hopkins. (2006). *Hormone Balance Made Simple.* New York: Grand Central Life & Style.

Wiley, T.S. and Bent Formby. (2000). *Lights Out: Sleep, Sugar, and Survival.* New York: Pocket Books.

Wilson, James L. (2001) Adrenal Fatigue: *The 21st Century Stress Syndrome.* Petaluma, CA: Smart Publications.

Young, D. Gary, N.D. (1996). *Aromatherapy: The Essential Beginning.* Salt Lake City, Utah: Essential Press Publishing.

Zavik, Jeffrey S. and Thompson, Jim. (2002). *Toxic Food Syndrome.* Ft. Lauderdale, FL: Fun Publishing.

CHAPTER 5

Cowan, L.D. et al. (1981, August). Breast Cancer Incidence in Women with a History of Progesterone Deficiency. *American Journal of Epidemiology,* 114 (2), 209-217.

FDA & HHS. (2009). Menopause and Hormones. Retrieved from http://www.fda.gov/forconsumers/byaudience/forwomen/ucm118624.htm.

Lee, John R., Jesse Hanley, and Virginia Hopkins. (1999). *What Your Doctor May Not Tell You about Pre-menopause.* New York: Grand Central Publishing.

Lee, John R. and Virginia Hopkins. (2004). *What Your Doctor May Not Tell You about Menopause.* New York: Wellness Central.

Lee, John R. and Virginia Hopkins. (2006). *Hormone Balance Made Simple.* New York: Grand Central Life & Style.

Maxson, W.S. (1987). The Use of Progesterone in the Treatment of PMS. *Clinical Obstetrics and Gynecology,* 30, 465-77.

Reiss, Uzzi. (2001). *Natural Hormone Balance for Women.* New York: Pocket Books.

Schwartz, Erika, M.D. (2002). *The Hormone Solution: Naturally Alleviate Symptoms of Hormone Imbalance from Adolescence through Menopause.* New York, NY: Warner Books.

Wiley, T.S. and Bent Formby. (2000). *Lights Out: Sleep, Sugar, and Survival*. New York: Pocket Books.

CHAPTER 6

Angell, Marcia. (2011, June 23). *The Epidemic of Mental Illness: Why? The New York Review of Books*.

Arntz, William, Chasse, Betsy & Vicente, Mark. (2005). *What the Bleep Do We Know!?* Deerfield Beach FL, Health Communications, Inc.

Brown, R., Kocsis, J.H., Caroff, S., Amsterdam, J., Winokur, A., Stokes, P.E. & Frazer, A. (1985). Differences in nocturnal melatonin secretion between melancholic Depressed patients and control subjects [Abstract]. *American Journal of Psychiatry*, 142, 811-816.

Chopra, Deepak. (1990). *Quantum Healing*. New York: Bantam Books.

Depression: Beyond Serotonin. (1999, March 1). *Psychology Today*. Retrieved from http://www.psychologytoday.com/print/22930.

Erdmann, Robert and Meirion Jones. (1995). *Fats that Can Save Your Life*.Port Orchard, WA: Bio-Science.

Hawkins, David R. (2002). *Power VS Force*. Carlsbad, Ca: Hay House Inc.

Hayes, Dave J. and Greenshaw, Andrew J. (2011). 5-HT receptors and reward-related behavior: A review. *Neuroscience and Biobehavioral Reviews*, 35, 1419-1449.

Kawai, Keisuke, Tamai, Hajime, Nishikata, Hiroaki, Kobayahi, Nobuyuke & Matsubayashi,Sunao. (1994). Severe Depression Associated with ACTH, PRL and GH Deficiency: A case Report. *Endocrine Journal*, 41(3), 275-79.

Kirsch, I. (2009). The Emperor's New Drugs: *Exploding the Antidepressant Myth*. London: The Bodley Head.

Krystal, John H., et al. (2011, Aug 3). Adjunctive Risperidone Treatment for Antidepressant-Resistant Symptoms of Chronic Military Service—Related PTSD. *JAMA, 306(5)*, 493-502.

Lee, John R. and Virginia Hopkins. (2006). *Hormone Balance Made Simple*. New York: Grand Central Life & Style.

Lyons, Philippa M., BSc. and Truswell, A. Stewart, M.D. (1988). Serotonin precursor influenced by type of carbohydrate meal in healthy adults. *Am J Clin Nutr*, 47, 433-39.

Ruller, Ray W. (1995, July/August). Neural Functions of Serotonin. *Science & Medicine*, 48-57.

Sheps, David S., MD, MSPH, Sheffield, David, PhD & Carney, Robert M., PhD. (1999). Does depression predict more symptoms or more disease? *Am Heart J*, 137, 386-7.

Wiley, T.S. and Bent Formby. (2000). *Lights Out: Sleep, Sugar, and Survival*. New York: Pocket Books.

Wilson, James L. (2001). Adrenal Fatigue: *The 21st Century Stress Syndrome*. Petaluma, CA: Smart Publications.

CHAPTER 7

Davis, Howard. (1998). *Feeling Younger with Homeopathic HGH*. Sheffield, MA: Safe Goods.

Elkins, Rita. (2004). *HGH: Age-Reversing Miracle*. Orem, UT: Woodland Publishing.

Klatz, Ronald & Kahn, Carol. (1997). *Grow Young with HGH*. New York: HarperCollinsPublishers Inc.

Weatherby, Dicken. (2005). *Naturally Raising Your HGH Levels*. Ashland, OR: Bear Mountain Publishing.

CHAPTER 8

Damian, Kate and Peter. (1995). *Aromatherpy Scent and Psyche.* Rochester, VT: Healing Arts Press.

Hay, Louise L. (1999). *You Can Heal Your Life.* Carlsbad, CA: Hay House, Inc.

Hirsch, Alan R. (1998). *Scentsational Weightloss.* New York: Fireside Books.

Hirsch, A.R., MD and Gomez, R. (1995). Weight Reduction Through Inhalation of Odorants. *J Neurol Med Surg*, 16, 28-31.

CHAPTER 9

Dr. Norman Orentreich, in his article: "Biology of Scalp Hair Growth," Clinics in Plastic Surgery -- Vol. 9, No. 2, 1982:

Yu. A. Vladimirov, A N Osipov, G I Klebanov (2003) Photobiological Principles of Therapeutic Applications of Laser Radiation.

Yu. A. Vladimirov, A N Osipov, G I Klebanov (2003) Photobiological Principles of Therapeutic Applications of Laser Radiation.

Women Hair Loss Council. "2009 Annual Report." 2009. Pdf file.

http://www.hlcconline.com/about-hair-loss.html

http://drbenkim.com/understanding-soft-tissue-injuries

http://www.ptbomassage.com/myofascial-release-wrinkle-treatment. html

RESOURCES

Saliva Hormone Testing

If you desire a full hormone saliva profile, please visit the following website to view the tests that they offer. Tests can be costly; however, this lab is high quality and affordable. While my clients do not often utilize tests, these particular saliva tests are a great way to scientifically show that your hormones are becoming balanced. Keep in mind that symptom alleviation is your final proof. Tests are not required before using any of the products or services on our website.

accessmedlabs.com

Brainwave Synchronization/"Sound-Wave" Therapy Audio CD's

This website offers a variety of relaxation that take brainwave patterns from a stressed Gamma/Beta wave all the way down to the slowest Delta wave—as mentioned in Chapter 8. Our local franchises offer the *Conditioned Response* program that includes this type of "sound-wave" therapy through our Becoming Balanced weight loss program. Their locations are listed on **bebalancedcenters.com.**

brainsync.com

Emotional Connection to your Physical Issue

It is always good to learn the emotional component to your specific ailments. Releasing the negative emotion associated with your condition will aid in your overall healing. The below book is a great reference for determining these connections.

You Can Heal Your Life by Louise L. Hay

Foods that Mesh with Your Blood Type

Although anyone can have a food sensitivity to wheat or dairy (or any other frequently consumed food), the differing blood types seem to have better results with certain foods and benefit from avoiding others. If you have consistent health issues, consider your diet as a possible contributing factor. The below book can help you to learn what foods to avoid and the ones that best suit you. This, as other tools, is simply a guide to help tweak your diet so it is perfect for you and your lifestyle.

Eat Right 4 Your Type by Peter J. D'Adamo and Catherine Whitney

Buffered Caffeine Coffee / Low Glycemic Sweetener

Daily use of these products, in place of regular caffeinated coffee, sugar and artificial sweeteners, will improve your overall mood, fat-burning potential and your long-term health. These products will aid in blood sugar stabilization and will help you to avoid insulin resistance (and diabetes), which increases hormonal imbalances.

boreshacoffee.com

Alkaline Water

This resource will aid you in alkalizing your water with an ionization machine in order to avoid estrogens found in plastic water bottles—all while also avoiding waste and saving money. Use of this type of water will improve alkalinity of the body, increase hydration of the body while fighting disease, and provide the body with antioxidants, which are infused into the water.

For a demonstration of how this system can reformulate your normal home tap water, go to **kangenwaterdemo.com**

Becoming Balanced...Hormonal Metabolic Correction Program

Our BeBalanced franchises offers the natural hormone balancing creams (***Pro Plus*** and ***Soothe Stress***), as well as the full Becoming Balanced weight loss program using the ketogenic/glandular protocol spoken of in Chapter 3 and 8. This unique protocol with proprietary supplements simultaneously aids in fast fat loss and hormone balancing. This program is offered through our BeBalanced franchise locations. See **bebalancedcenters.com** for local listing. The website also offers a free online hormone assessment which includes a natural hormone balancing specialist following up with you to go over your results.

CPSIA information can be obtained
at www.ICGtesting.com
Printed in the USA
JSHW011450150819
1084JS00002B/4